Empowering Your Prostate Health

Nonsurgical Strategies for Overcoming Prostate Cancer

By

Calvin M. Duncan

Table Of Contents

INTRODUCTION

Understanding the Prostate

The prostate gland, a small but vital organ in the male reproductive system, plays a crucial role in maintaining a man's sexual and urinary health. In this comprehensive exploration, we will delve into the intricate details of the prostate, from its anatomy and function to its importance in overall well-being. By the end of this discussion, you will have a profound understanding of the prostate and its significance in men's lives.

The prostate gland is a walnut-sized organ situated just below the bladder, encircling the upper part of the urethra, the tube responsible for transporting urine and semen out of the body. While it may be small in size, its functions are pivotal to male reproductive and urinary health.

Anatomy of the Prostate

To comprehend the role and importance of the prostate, it's essential to grasp its anatomical structure. The prostate is composed of several key components:

1. Lobes: The prostate gland is divided into lobes, with the most commonly referred to being the anterior, posterior, and lateral lobes. These divisions help in anatomical and diagnostic descriptions of the gland.

2. Zones: The prostate is further categorized into zones, including the peripheral zone, central zone, and transitional zone. Each zone has distinct characteristics and plays different roles in prostate function.

3. Ducts and Glands: The prostate consists of numerous small glands and ducts that produce and transport seminal fluid. These fluids contribute to the nourishment, protection, and transport of sperm during ejaculation.

4. Muscles and Connective Tissue: Muscles and connective tissue surround the prostate, helping to support its structure and function. These elements play a role in the ejaculation process.

Function of the Prostate

The primary function of the prostate gland is to secrete seminal fluid, a key component of semen. Seminal fluid serves several critical roles in the male reproductive process:

1. Nutrient Supply: Seminal fluid provides nutrients and energy to sperm, enhancing their ability to move and survive.

2. Sperm Protection: It protects sperm from the acidic environment of the male urethra and the female reproductive tract, increasing their chances of reaching and fertilizing an egg.

3. Sperm Transport: Seminal fluid helps transport sperm through the urethra and into the female reproductive tract during ejaculation.

4. Lubrication: It contributes to the lubrication of the urethra and facilitates the passage of semen during ejaculation.

5. Neutralizing Acidity: Seminal fluid neutralizes the acidic environment of the vagina, creating a more favorable environment for sperm survival.

The Importance of the Prostate

The prostate gland holds immense importance in a man's life, impacting both sexual and urinary health. Its significance can be categorized into the following aspects:

1. Reproductive Health: The prostate's role in semen production and sperm transport is fundamental for male fertility. Without the prostate's contribution, the chances of successful fertilization would be significantly reduced.

2. Ejaculation: The prostate plays a key role in the ejaculation process. During sexual arousal, the prostate contracts to expel seminal fluid into the urethra, which is then ejected from the body during ejaculation. This process is vital for sexual satisfaction and reproduction.

3. Urinary Health: While primarily associated with reproductive function, the prostate's location and size can impact urinary health. In some cases, an enlarged prostate can obstruct the flow of urine, leading to urinary symptoms such as frequent urination, difficulty starting and stopping urine flow, and nocturia (nighttime urination).

4. Prostate-Specific Antigen (PSA) Production: The prostate is responsible for producing prostate-specific antigen (PSA), a protein that can be measured through a blood test. PSA levels are used in prostate cancer screening and monitoring, making it a crucial biomarker for early detection and management of prostate cancer.

Prostate Health and Age

As men age, the prostate undergoes changes that can affect its size and function. One common age-related condition affecting the prostate is benign prostatic hyperplasia (BPH), which is the non-cancerous enlargement of the prostate gland. BPH is a prevalent condition in older men and can lead to urinary symptoms such as urinary frequency, urgency, and weak urine flow.

Another age-related concern is prostate cancer, which becomes more prevalent with advancing age. Prostate cancer is a significant health issue for older men, and understanding the prostate's role and behavior is essential for early detection and treatment.

Prostate-Related Conditions

Several conditions and diseases can affect the prostate gland, ranging from benign to malignant. Understanding these conditions is crucial for managing prostate health effectively.

1. Benign Prostatic Hyperplasia (BPH): BPH, also known as prostate gland enlargement, is a non-cancerous condition where the prostate increases in size, causing symptoms related to urinary flow obstruction. It is a common condition in older men and can be managed through medications or surgical interventions.

2. Prostatitis: Prostatitis is the inflammation of the prostate gland and can result from infection or other causes. It often leads to symptoms such as pelvic pain, urinary difficulties, and discomfort. Treatment depends on the underlying cause and may involve antibiotics or anti-inflammatory medications.

3. Prostate Cancer: Prostate cancer is the most concerning prostate-related condition. It occurs when cells in the prostate gland mutate and multiply uncontrollably, forming a tumor. Prostate cancer is the second most common cancer in men globally and requires prompt diagnosis and treatment to maximize survival rates.

Prostate Cancer: Understanding the Enemy

Prostate cancer is a type of cancer that affects the prostate gland in men. The prostate gland is a small, walnut-shaped organ located below the bladder and in front of the rectum. It is responsible for producing semen, the fluid that carries sperm.

When prostate cells start to grow and divide uncontrollably, it can lead to the formation of a tumor. While some prostate tumors are benign (non-cancerous) and do not spread to other parts of the body, others can be malignant (cancerous) and have the potential to spread to nearby tissues and organs.

Prostate cancer is one of the most common types of cancer in men, especially in older age. It usually develops slowly over time and may not cause noticeable symptoms in its early stages.

However, as the cancer progresses, symptoms such as difficulty urinating, blood in the urine or semen, erectile dysfunction, and pain in the pelvic area may occur.

Risk Factors for Prostate Cancer

Understanding the risk factors associated with prostate cancer is crucial for identifying individuals who may be at a higher risk of developing the disease. While prostate cancer can affect anyone, certain factors increase the likelihood of its occurrence:

1. Age: Age is the most significant risk factor for prostate cancer. The risk increases substantially after the age of 50, with the majority of cases diagnosed in men over 65.

2. Family History: A family history of prostate cancer, especially in close relatives like a father or brother, can elevate an individual's risk.

3. Race and Ethnicity: Prostate cancer incidence varies among racial and ethnic groups. African American men have a higher risk of developing prostate cancer, and they are also more likely to develop aggressive forms of the disease.

4. Genetic Mutations: Inherited mutations in certain genes, such as BRCA1 and BRCA2, are associated with an increased risk of prostate cancer. These mutations are also linked to breast and ovarian cancer.

5. Diet and Lifestyle: While the relationship between diet and prostate cancer is still being studied, a diet high in red meat and dairy products and low in fruits and vegetables may be associated with a higher risk. Obesity and a sedentary lifestyle are also considered potential risk factors.

6. Geographic Location: Prostate cancer incidence varies by geographic location, with higher rates in North America and Western Europe and lower rates in Asia. Lifestyle and dietary factors may contribute to these differences.

Prostate Cancer Screening and Diagnosis

Early detection is critical for effectively managing prostate cancer and improving outcomes. Several screening and diagnostic methods are available to assess the presence and extent of prostate cancer:

1. Digital Rectal Examination (DRE): During a DRE, a healthcare provider inserts a gloved, lubricated finger into the rectum to feel for any abnormalities or irregularities in the prostate gland. While not a definitive diagnostic tool, it can raise suspicion and prompt further evaluation.

2. Prostate-Specific Antigen (PSA) Test: The PSA test measures the level of PSA, a protein produced by the prostate gland, in the blood. Elevated PSA levels can indicate various prostate conditions, including cancer. However, an elevated PSA level does not necessarily indicate cancer, and further testing is typically needed for a definitive diagnosis.

3. Biopsy: If elevated PSA levels or abnormal DRE results raise suspicion of prostate cancer, a biopsy is typically performed. This involves the removal of small tissue samples from the prostate gland for examination under a microscope. Biopsy results provide information about the presence, grade, and extent of cancer.

4. Imaging Studies: Advanced imaging techniques such as MRI, CT scans, and bone scans may be used to assess the extent of cancer spread, especially in advanced stages.

Understanding PSA Levels

Prostate-specific antigen (PSA) is a protein produced by the prostate gland. It is normally present in small amounts in the blood, but elevated PSA levels can be indicative of various prostate conditions, including cancer. However, interpreting PSA levels requires careful consideration, as several factors can influence them.

Normal PSA Levels:

PSA levels below 4 nanograms per milliliter (ng/mL) are generally considered normal. However, some men with prostate cancer may have PSA levels within this range.

Elevated PSA Levels:

PSA levels between 4 and 10 ng/mL may be considered mildly elevated, and further evaluation is typically recommended. PSA levels above 10 ng/mL are more concerning and often warrant additional testing.

Factors Influencing PSA Levels:

 PSA levels can be influenced by age, prostate size, medications, and certain medical conditions. It is essential to consider these factors when interpreting PSA test results.

Grading and Staging of Prostate Cancer

Once prostate cancer is diagnosed, it is important to determine its grade and stage, which provide critical information for treatment planning and prognosis.

1. Gleason Score: Prostate cancer is typically graded using the Gleason score, a system developed by pathologist Dr. Donald Gleason. This system assigns a score ranging from 2 to 10 based on the appearance of cancer cells under a microscope. Higher scores indicate more aggressive cancer. The Gleason score helps categorize prostate cancer into different grades, providing insights into its behavior.

2. TNM Staging: Prostate cancer is also staged using the TNM system, which evaluates the size and extent of the primary tumor (T), whether cancer has spread to nearby lymph nodes (N), and whether there are distant metastases (M). This system helps categorize prostate cancer into stages ranging from I (localized) to IV (advanced).

Stage I: Cancer is confined to the prostate gland and is usually small and slow-growing.

Stage II: Cancer remains within the prostate gland but may be larger or more aggressive than in Stage I.

Stage III: Cancer has extended beyond the prostate capsule and may involve nearby tissues or seminal vesicles.

Stage IV: Cancer has spread to distant sites in the body, such as bones or lymph nodes, indicating advanced disease.

Treatment Options for Prostate Cancer

The choice of treatment for prostate cancer depends on various factors, including the stage and grade of the cancer, the age and overall health of the patient, and the patient's preferences. Treatment options for prostate cancer can be broadly categorized into the following:

1. Active Surveillance: For low-risk prostate cancer, active surveillance may be recommended. This approach involves closely monitoring the cancer with regular check-ups, biopsies, and imaging, with the option of initiating treatment if the cancer shows signs of progression.

2. Surgery: Prostatectomy, the surgical removal of the prostate gland, is a common treatment for localized prostate cancer. There are different surgical techniques, including open surgery and minimally invasive approaches such as laparoscopic or robotic-assisted surgery.

3. Radiation Therapy: Radiation therapy uses high-energy rays to target and kill cancer cells. It can be delivered externally (external beam radiation) or internally (brachytherapy), depending on the patient's specific situation.

4. Hormone Therapy: Also known as androgen deprivation therapy (ADT), hormone therapy aims to reduce the levels of male hormones (androgens) in the body, as these hormones can fuel the growth of prostate cancer cells.

5. Chemotherapy: Chemotherapy is typically reserved for advanced or metastatic prostate cancer. It involves the use of drugs to kill cancer cells throughout the body.

6. Immunotherapy: Immunotherapy is an emerging treatment option that harnesses the body's immune system to target and attack cancer cells. It is being studied as a potential therapy for prostate cancer.

7. Targeted Therapies: Targeted therapies are drugs that specifically target molecules or pathways involved in cancer growth and progression. They are sometimes used in combination with other treatments.

8. Clinical Trials: Participation in clinical trials can provide access to cutting-edge treatments and therapies that are still in the experimental stage.

Side Effects and Quality of Life

Each prostate cancer treatment option comes with its own set of potential side effects, which can impact a patient's quality of life. For example, surgery can lead to urinary incontinence and erectile dysfunction, while radiation therapy may cause urinary and bowel problems. Hormone therapy can result in hot flashes, fatigue, and changes in sexual function.

Shared Decision-Making

Deciding on the most appropriate treatment for prostate cancer is a complex and deeply personal process. It often involves shared decision-making between the patient and their healthcare team. Patients should actively participate in discussions about treatment options, potential side effects, and expected outcomes to make choices aligned with their values and goals.

Understanding the prostate gland, its function, and its role in health and disease is paramount for all men. The prostate is not just a walnut-sized organ; it is a key player in both reproductive and urinary health. From semen production to ejaculation and its involvement in prostate cancer, the prostate has a profound impact on a man's life.

Prostate-related conditions, including benign prostatic hyperplasia (BPH), prostatitis, and prostate cancer, are complex and require careful consideration. Early detection, through methods like the PSA test and digital rectal examination, is essential for managing these conditions effectively.

Prostate cancer, in particular, necessitates a deep understanding to make informed decisions about screening, diagnosis, and treatment. From risk factors and grading to staging and treatment options, the journey through prostate cancer requires both medical expertise and active patient involvement.

In conclusion, the prostate is not just an organ; it is a symbol of masculinity, fertility, and vitality. Understanding its intricacies empowers men to take charge of their health and well-being, ensuring that they can continue to lead fulfilling lives with confidence and dignity.

The Importance of Nonsurgical Approaches

While surgery is a commonly employed treatment option for prostate cancer, nonsurgical approaches have gained increasing importance in recent years. These approaches encompass a range of therapies and strategies that offer both curative and palliative benefits, often with fewer associated side effects and a better quality of life for patients. In this comprehensive discussion, we will delve into the various nonsurgical approaches used in the management of prostate cancer, emphasizing their importance and the advantages they bring to patients.

While surgery remains a vital tool in the arsenal against this disease, there is growing recognition of the importance of nonsurgical approaches in treating prostate cancer.

Nonsurgical approaches encompass a wide range of strategies and therapies, including radiation therapy, hormonal therapy, chemotherapy, immunotherapy, targeted therapies, active surveillance, and watchful waiting. These approaches offer various advantages, such as preserving quality of life, minimizing side effects, and tailoring treatment to the individual patient's needs and the stage of their cancer. This discussion will explore each of these nonsurgical approaches and emphasize their significance in prostate cancer care.

Radiation Therapy

Radiation therapy is a cornerstone of nonsurgical prostate cancer treatment. It involves the use of high-energy rays, such as X-rays or protons, to target and kill cancer cells. Radiation therapy can be administered in two primary forms: external beam radiation and brachytherapy.

- External Beam Radiation: External beam radiation therapy delivers radiation from outside the body, precisely targeting the prostate gland. It is typically administered over several weeks, with daily treatments lasting only a few minutes each. External beam radiation is highly effective in treating localized prostate cancer, with curative intent.
- Brachytherapy: Brachytherapy, also known as seed implantation, involves the placement of radioactive seeds directly into the prostate gland. These seeds emit radiation locally, targeting the cancer cells while minimizing exposure to surrounding healthy tissues. Brachytherapy is an effective treatment option, particularly for low-risk and intermediate-risk prostate cancer.

Advantages of Radiation Therapy:

- Non-invasive: Radiation therapy does not require surgical incisions, reducing the risk of complications and infections.

- Preserves anatomical integrity: Radiation therapy aims to preserve the structure and function of the prostate gland.

- Minimal recovery time: Patients can typically resume their daily activities shortly after each radiation treatment session.

Hormonal Therapy

Hormonal therapy, also known as androgen deprivation therapy (ADT), is a nonsurgical approach that aims to reduce the levels of male hormones, primarily testosterone, in the body. Since prostate cancer growth is often dependent on testosterone, hormonal therapy can be an effective way to slow the progression of the disease.

Hormonal therapy can be administered through various methods, including injections, oral medications, or surgical removal of the testicles (orchiectomy). It is often used in combination with other treatments for prostate cancer, such as radiation therapy or chemotherapy.

Advantages of Hormonal Therapy:

- Effective control: Hormonal therapy can effectively control the growth of prostate cancer, particularly in advanced or metastatic cases.

- Few immediate side effects: Compared to surgery, hormonal therapy typically has fewer immediate side effects.

- Non-invasive: Hormonal therapy does not require surgery, making it a preferred choice for some patients.

Chemotherapy

Chemotherapy involves the use of drugs to target and kill rapidly dividing cancer cells throughout the body. While it is not typically the first-line treatment for localized prostate cancer, it can be an essential part of the treatment plan for advanced or metastatic disease.

Advantages of Chemotherapy:

- Systemic treatment: Chemotherapy targets cancer cells that may have spread to other parts of the body, making it suitable for advanced cases.

- Palliative care: In advanced prostate cancer, chemotherapy can help alleviate symptoms and improve the patient's quality of life.

Immunotherapy

Immunotherapy is an emerging and promising approach in cancer treatment. It harnesses the body's immune system to recognize and target cancer cells. While it is still being studied in the context of prostate cancer, immunotherapy has shown potential as a treatment option.

Immunotherapies such as sipuleucel-T (Provenge) have been approved for the treatment of advanced prostate cancer. These therapies involve extracting immune cells from the patient, modifying them to target prostate cancer cells, and then infusing them back into the patient.

Advantages of Immunotherapy:

- Targeted treatment: Immunotherapy specifically targets cancer cells, minimizing damage to healthy tissues.

- Potential for long-term remission: Some immunotherapies have shown the potential to induce durable responses in advanced prostate cancer.

Targeted Therapies

Targeted therapies are drugs that specifically target molecules or pathways involved in cancer growth and progression. They are designed to disrupt specific mechanisms that cancer cells use to thrive. Targeted therapies are often used in combination with other treatments.

Advantages of Targeted Therapies:

- Precision medicine: Targeted therapies are tailored to the specific characteristics of the patient's cancer, potentially improving treatment effectiveness.

- Reduced side effects: By specifically targeting cancer cells, these therapies may result in fewer side effects than traditional chemotherapy.

Active Surveillance

Active surveillance is an approach that involves closely monitoring the progression of prostate cancer in patients with low-risk or very low-risk disease. Instead of immediate treatment, active surveillance focuses on regular check-ups, PSA tests, digital rectal examinations, and periodic biopsies to track the cancer's behavior.

Advantages of Active Surveillance:

- Preserves quality of life: Active surveillance allows patients to avoid the potential side effects of unnecessary treatment.

- Individualized approach: Treatment decisions can be tailored to the patient's unique situation, reducing overtreatment.

Watchful Waiting

Watchful waiting is a more passive approach to prostate cancer management, typically chosen for older individuals or those with multiple serious health conditions. Unlike active surveillance, watchful waiting does not involve routine biopsies or aggressive monitoring. Instead, it focuses on managing symptoms as they arise.

Advantages of Watchful Waiting:

- Minimizes interventions: Watchful waiting is often chosen to avoid the potential complications of aggressive treatment in patients with limited life expectancy.

- Quality of life: It prioritizes the patient's comfort and quality of life, emphasizing symptom management over aggressive treatment.

The Importance of Nonsurgical Approaches

The importance of nonsurgical approaches in the management of prostate cancer cannot be overstated. These approaches offer several critical advantages that contribute to the well-being of patients:

1. Preserving Quality of Life: Nonsurgical approaches, such as radiation therapy and hormonal therapy, aim to preserve the quality of life by minimizing the potential side effects associated with surgery. This includes preserving urinary and sexual function, which can be significantly impacted by surgery.

2. Tailoring Treatment: Nonsurgical approaches allow for individualized treatment plans based on the patient's cancer stage, risk factors, and overall health. This tailored approach helps avoid overtreatment in low-risk cases and ensures aggressive treatment for high-risk or advanced disease.

3. Combination Therapies: Many nonsurgical approaches can be used in combination with one another or with surgery to optimize treatment outcomes. For example, radiation therapy and hormonal therapy are often combined to increase treatment effectiveness.

4. Minimizing Invasiveness: Nonsurgical approaches are generally less invasive than surgery, reducing the risk of complications, infections, and lengthy recovery periods.

5. Palliative Care: In advanced or metastatic prostate cancer, nonsurgical approaches such as chemotherapy and immunotherapy provide palliative care, improving symptoms and enhancing the patient's quality of life.

6. Advancements in Research: Research in nonsurgical approaches, particularly immunotherapy and targeted therapies, is ongoing and holds promise for more effective treatments in the future.

Prostate cancer is a complex and multifaceted disease that requires a diverse range of treatment options. While surgery remains an important tool in the fight against prostate cancer, the significance of nonsurgical approaches cannot be understated. These approaches, including radiation therapy, hormonal therapy, chemotherapy, immunotherapy, targeted therapies, active surveillance, and watchful waiting, offer patients a range of benefits, from preserving quality of life to tailoring treatment to the individual's unique situation.

The importance of nonsurgical approaches is not only evident in their ability to effectively treat prostate cancer but also in their capacity to improve the overall well-being of patients. As medical research continues to advance, these approaches will play an increasingly vital role in prostate cancer care, offering hope and improved outcomes for countless individuals affected by this disease.

CHAPTER ONE

Screening for Prostate Cancer: Balancing Benefits and Risks

Screening for prostate cancer is a critical tool in early detection and treatment. However, the topic of screening is complex, as it involves a delicate balance between the benefits of early detection and the potential harms of overdiagnosis and overtreatment. In this comprehensive discussion, we will explore the key aspects of prostate cancer screening, including the methods used, the controversies surrounding it, and the importance of informed decision-making.

Screening for prostate cancer aims to detect the disease at an early, treatable stage when curative interventions are most effective. Two primary methods are commonly used for prostate cancer screening: the prostate-specific antigen (PSA) test and digital rectal examination (DRE).

The PSA Test

The PSA test measures the level of prostate-specific antigen, a protein produced by the prostate gland, in the blood. Elevated PSA levels can be indicative of various prostate conditions, including cancer. The test is relatively simple, involving a blood draw, and is widely available.

Digital Rectal Examination (DRE)

During a DRE, a healthcare provider inserts a gloved, lubricated finger into the rectum to feel for any abnormalities or irregularities in the prostate gland. While not a definitive diagnostic tool, it can raise suspicion and prompt further evaluation.

Benefits of Prostate Cancer Screening

1. Early Detection: The primary benefit of prostate cancer screening is the potential for early detection, allowing for timely treatment and improved outcomes. When prostate cancer is diagnosed at an early stage, it is more likely to be curable.

2. Reduction in Mortality: Studies have suggested that prostate cancer screening can lead to a reduction in prostate cancer-related mortality. Detecting and treating aggressive cancers early can prevent their progression to advanced, incurable stages.

3. Increased Treatment Options: Early detection provides patients with a broader range of treatment options, including less invasive therapies and the potential for cure.

4. Peace of Mind: Regular screening can provide peace of mind for men concerned about their prostate health. Knowing their PSA levels and prostate health status can alleviate anxiety.

Controversies and Challenges

Despite the potential benefits, prostate cancer screening is a topic fraught with controversies and challenges. These stem from several key issues:

1. Overdiagnosis: One of the most significant concerns with prostate cancer screening is the risk of overdiagnosis. This occurs when screening detects slow-growing cancers that would never have caused symptoms or harm during a person's lifetime. Overdiagnosis can lead to unnecessary treatments with potential side effects.

2. Overtreatment: Overdiagnosis often leads to overtreatment, where patients undergo aggressive interventions such as surgery or radiation therapy for cancers that may not have required treatment. Overtreatment can result in significant physical and psychological consequences.

3. False Positives and False Negatives: The PSA test and DRE are not perfect, and they can yield false-positive or false-negative results. False positives can lead to unnecessary anxiety and biopsies, while false negatives can provide a false sense of security.

4. Uncertainty in Risk Assessment: Assessing an individual's risk of aggressive prostate cancer accurately is challenging. Some men with elevated PSA levels may have indolent cancers, while others with normal PSA levels may have aggressive disease.

5. Age and Life Expectancy: Decisions about prostate cancer screening should consider a man's age and life expectancy. Screening may not be appropriate for older individuals with limited life expectancy, as the potential benefits may not outweigh the risks.

Informed Decision-Making

Given the complexities and controversies surrounding prostate cancer screening, informed decision-making is essential. Men considering screening should be fully informed about the benefits and risks to make decisions aligned with their values and preferences. Key aspects of informed decision-making include:

1. Understanding the Risks: Men should be aware of the risk of overdiagnosis, overtreatment, and potential side effects of treatments such as surgery or radiation therapy.

2. Shared Decision-Making: Healthcare providers should engage in shared decision-making with patients, discussing the pros and cons of screening and helping patients make choices aligned with their individual circumstances.

3. Individualized Screening: Screening decisions should be individualized based on factors such as age, family history, overall health, and personal preferences.

4. Active Surveillance: For men at low risk of aggressive prostate cancer, active surveillance may be an appropriate alternative to immediate treatment. This approach involves close monitoring and intervention only if the cancer shows signs of progression.

5. Discussion of Treatment Options: In the event of a positive screening result, patients should have a thorough discussion with their healthcare providers about treatment options, potential side effects, and the likely outcomes.

Prostate cancer screening is a double-edged sword, offering the potential benefits of early detection and reduced mortality while carrying the risks of overdiagnosis and overtreatment. The decision to undergo screening should be based on informed choices that consider an individual's risk factors, values, and preferences. Healthcare providers play a crucial role in guiding patients through the decision-making process, providing clear information about the benefits and risks of screening.

Ultimately, the importance of prostate cancer screening lies in its potential to save lives through early detection and intervention. However, the decision to screen should not be taken lightly, as it requires a nuanced understanding of the complexities and controversies surrounding prostate cancer and its management. Informed decision-making empowers individuals to take charge of their health while minimizing the potential harms associated with screening and treatment.

PSA Testing: Pros and Cons in Prostate Health

Prostate-specific antigen (PSA) testing is a commonly used tool for prostate cancer screening and monitoring. It has been instrumental in the early detection of prostate cancer, helping to identify cases at a treatable stage. However, the use of PSA testing is not without controversy and drawbacks. In this comprehensive discussion, we will explore the pros and cons of PSA testing, emphasizing its role in prostate health and the importance of informed decision-making.

The PSA Test: What Is It?

The PSA test measures the level of prostate-specific antigen (PSA), a protein produced by the prostate gland, in the blood. PSA is normally present in small amounts in the bloodstream, but elevated levels can indicate various prostate conditions, including cancer.

The Pros of PSA Testing

1. Early Detection: The primary advantage of PSA testing is its potential to detect prostate cancer at an early, treatable stage. Early detection often leads to more successful treatment outcomes, as the cancer is less likely to have spread beyond the prostate gland.

2. Reduction in Mortality: Numerous studies have suggested that PSA testing can lead to a reduction in prostate cancer-related mortality. Detecting and treating aggressive cancers early can prevent their progression to advanced, incurable stages.

3. Treatment Options: When prostate cancer is diagnosed at an early stage, patients have a broader range of treatment options, including less invasive therapies such as radiation therapy or active surveillance.

4. Monitoring Prostate Health: PSA testing is not limited to cancer detection. It can also be used to monitor the overall health of the prostate, helping to identify changes over time.

5. Risk Stratification: PSA levels can help risk-stratify patients. Individuals with consistently low PSA levels may have a lower risk of aggressive prostate cancer and may require less frequent screening.

The Cons of PSA Testing

1. Risk of Overdiagnosis: One of the most significant drawbacks of PSA testing is the risk of overdiagnosis. Overdiagnosis occurs when screening detects slow-growing cancers that would never have caused symptoms or harm during a person's lifetime. This can lead to unnecessary treatments with potential side effects.

2. Overtreatment: Overdiagnosis often leads to overtreatment, where patients undergo aggressive interventions such as surgery or radiation therapy for cancers that may not have required treatment. Overtreatment can result in significant physical and psychological consequences.

3. False Positives and False Negatives: The PSA test is not infallible and can yield false-positive or false-negative results. False positives can lead to unnecessary anxiety and biopsies, while false negatives can provide a false sense of security.

4. Uncertainty in Risk Assessment: Assessing an individual's risk of aggressive prostate cancer accurately is challenging. Some men with elevated PSA levels may have indolent cancers, while others with normal PSA levels may have aggressive disease.

5. Age and Life Expectancy: Decisions about PSA testing should consider a man's age and life expectancy. Screening may not be appropriate for older individuals with limited life expectancy, as the potential benefits may not outweigh the risks.

The Evolving Role of PSA Testing

In recent years, there has been a shift in the approach to PSA testing. Instead of routine, widespread screening, healthcare providers are increasingly emphasizing shared decision-making and individualized screening based on risk factors and patient preferences. This approach aims to maximize the benefits of early detection while minimizing the risks of overdiagnosis and overtreatment.

Additionally, research continues to explore ways to improve the accuracy of PSA testing and refine risk assessment. Newer methods, such as the use of PSA density, PSA velocity, and risk calculators, are being investigated to enhance the precision of screening and reduce the likelihood of false positives.

PSA testing is a valuable tool in prostate health that has played a significant role in the early detection of prostate cancer. However, its use is not without controversy and drawbacks, primarily related to the risk of overdiagnosis and overtreatment. Informed decision-making is essential for men considering PSA testing, as it allows them to weigh the potential benefits of early detection against the risks of unnecessary treatment.

The evolving approach to PSA testing emphasizes individualized screening, shared decision-making, and ongoing research to refine risk assessment. Ultimately, the goal is to maximize the benefits of PSA testing while minimizing its potential harms, ensuring that men can make informed choices about their prostate health based on their unique circumstances and preferences.

Digital Rectal Examination (DRE)

The digital rectal examination (DRE) is a vital and time-tested component of prostate health evaluation. It is a physical examination conducted by a healthcare provider to assess the condition of the prostate gland, located just below the bladder and in front of the rectum. While the DRE may not be as widely discussed as the prostate-specific antigen (PSA) blood test, it plays a crucial role in detecting prostate abnormalities, including cancer, and provides valuable information for diagnosis and treatment decisions. In this comprehensive exploration, we will delve into the various aspects of the DRE, its significance in prostate health, the procedure itself, and its role in the broader context of prostate cancer screening and assessment.

The Role of Digital Rectal Examination (DRE)

The DRE is a physical examination performed by a healthcare provider, typically a urologist or primary care physician. During the examination, the healthcare provider inserts a gloved, lubricated finger into the patient's rectum to assess the condition of the prostate gland. The DRE serves several essential purposes in prostate health evaluation:

1. Detecting Abnormalities: The primary goal of the DRE is to detect abnormalities in the prostate gland. These abnormalities can include changes in size, shape, texture, or the presence of nodules or masses. The DRE can raise suspicion of prostate conditions that warrant further investigation, including prostate cancer.

2. Assessing Prostate Size: The DRE allows the healthcare provider to assess the size of the prostate gland. An enlarged prostate, a condition known as benign prostatic hyperplasia (BPH), can cause urinary symptoms such as frequent urination, urgency, and weak urine flow. Assessing prostate size is essential in diagnosing and managing BPH.

3. Evaluating Prostate Texture: The DRE provides information about the texture of the prostate. A normal prostate is typically smooth and rubbery. Changes in texture, such as hardness or irregularity, may be indicative of prostate abnormalities, including cancer.

4. Guiding Biopsy: If the DRE raises suspicion of prostate cancer, the healthcare provider may recommend a prostate biopsy. The DRE helps guide the biopsy needle to target specific areas of concern within the prostate gland, allowing for the collection of tissue samples for laboratory analysis.

5. Monitoring Disease Progression: For men already diagnosed with prostate conditions, such as prostate cancer or BPH, the DRE is used to monitor disease progression and treatment effectiveness over time.

6. Baseline Assessment: Establishing a baseline DRE can be valuable for future comparisons. If changes occur in the prostate gland, a series of DREs can help track these changes and guide further evaluation and treatment decisions.

The Digital Rectal Examination Procedure

The DRE procedure involves several key steps:

1. Preparation: Before the examination, the patient may be asked to change into a hospital gown or remove clothing from the waist down. The patient then lies on their side with their knees drawn toward their chest or bends forward over an examination table.

2. Glove and Lubrication: The healthcare provider wears a lubricated glove on one hand. The lubrication is essential for minimizing discomfort and allowing the healthcare provider's finger to glide smoothly into the rectum.

3. Insertion and Examination: The healthcare provider gently inserts their lubricated, gloved finger into the patient's rectum. They use their finger to feel the prostate gland, which is located just a few inches inside the rectum. The examination typically lasts only a few seconds.

4. Assessment: During the examination, the healthcare provider assesses the size, shape, texture, and any abnormalities of the prostate gland. Any areas of concern, such as nodules or hardness, are noted.

5. Conclusion: After completing the examination, the healthcare provider removes their gloved finger and discusses their findings with the patient. They may provide immediate feedback or schedule additional tests or consultations based on their observations.

Benefits and Limitations of the Digital Rectal Examination

The DRE offers several benefits in prostate health evaluation:

1. Complementary to PSA Testing: The DRE complements other screening methods, such as the PSA blood test. While the PSA test measures the level of a specific protein in the blood, the DRE provides a physical assessment of the prostate gland, allowing for a more comprehensive evaluation.

2. Immediate Assessment: The DRE provides immediate information to the healthcare provider during the examination, allowing for prompt evaluation and potential recommendations for further testing or treatment.

3. Guidance for Biopsy: If the DRE raises suspicion of prostate cancer, it can guide the healthcare provider in performing a prostate biopsy, which is the definitive diagnostic test for prostate cancer.

However, the DRE also has limitations:

1. Subjective Assessment: The DRE relies on the healthcare provider's subjective assessment of the prostate gland's size, texture, and abnormalities. Interpretation can vary among providers, and the examination may miss subtle abnormalities.

2. Limited Detection: The DRE may not detect early-stage prostate cancer, particularly in cases where cancerous changes are small or localized deep within the gland.

3. Discomfort: Some men may find the DRE uncomfortable or embarrassing. However, it is generally a quick and well-tolerated procedure.

4. Inconclusive Findings: In some cases, the DRE may yield inconclusive findings, necessitating further tests, such as a prostate biopsy, for a definitive diagnosis.

Role of the DRE in Prostate Cancer Screening

Prostate cancer screening typically involves a combination of the DRE and PSA testing. The DRE can detect abnormalities that may not be reflected in PSA levels alone, making it a valuable tool in early detection. However, it is essential to recognize that the DRE is not a standalone diagnostic test for prostate cancer.

The DRE's role in prostate cancer screening and assessment includes:

1. Risk Assessment: The DRE helps assess a man's risk of prostate cancer by identifying physical abnormalities or changes in the prostate gland that may warrant further investigation.

2. Early Detection: The DRE can aid in the early detection of prostate cancer, particularly when it is accompanied by other screening methods such as PSA testing.

3. Guidance for Biopsy: If the DRE raises suspicion of prostate cancer, it can guide the healthcare provider in performing a prostate biopsy to collect tissue samples for laboratory analysis.

4. Monitoring: For men with known prostate cancer, the DRE is used to monitor the progression of the disease and the effectiveness of treatment.

The digital rectal examination (DRE) is a valuable and time-tested component of prostate health evaluation. While it may not be as widely discussed as the PSA blood test, the DRE plays a crucial role in detecting prostate abnormalities, including cancer, and provides valuable information for diagnosis and treatment decisions. When used in conjunction with other screening methods and in the context of informed decision-making, the DRE contributes to the early detection and management of prostate conditions, ultimately promoting the well-being and prostate health of men worldwide.

Advanced Diagnostic Techniques for Prostate Cancer

Prostate cancer is a complex and prevalent disease that affects millions of men worldwide. Early detection and accurate diagnosis are crucial for effective treatment and improved outcomes. While traditional diagnostic methods, such as the prostate-specific antigen (PSA) test and digital rectal examination (DRE), remain important, advanced diagnostic techniques have emerged in recent years, revolutionizing the way prostate cancer is detected, characterized, and managed. In this comprehensive discussion, we will explore the advanced diagnostic techniques used in the assessment of prostate cancer, emphasizing their significance, advantages, limitations, and their role in personalized treatment strategies.

Advanced diagnostic techniques have emerged to address these challenges, providing more accurate and personalized information about prostate cancer.

1. Multiparametric Magnetic Resonance Imaging (mpMRI)

Multiparametric magnetic resonance imaging (mpMRI) is a non-invasive imaging technique that has revolutionized the detection and characterization of prostate cancer. It combines several MRI sequences to provide a comprehensive view of the prostate gland, enabling the identification of suspicious areas for targeted biopsy. The key components of mpMRI include:

- T2-Weighted Imaging: This sequence provides high-resolution anatomical images of the prostate, allowing for the visualization of abnormalities, such as tumors, within the gland.

- Diffusion-Weighted Imaging (DWI): DWI measures the movement of water molecules in tissues. In prostate cancer, areas with restricted water diffusion are indicative of malignancy.

- Dynamic Contrast-Enhanced Imaging (DCE): DCE involves the injection of a contrast agent to assess blood flow in the prostate. Cancerous tissues typically exhibit increased vascularity.

- Proton Magnetic Resonance Spectroscopy (MRS): MRS provides information about the metabolic activity of tissues. Elevated levels of certain metabolites can suggest the presence of cancer.

Advantages of mpMRI:

- Improved Detection: mpMRI can detect prostate cancer lesions that may be missed by traditional methods, reducing the risk of false negatives.

- Targeted Biopsies: Suspicious areas identified on mpMRI can be precisely targeted during biopsy procedures, improving the accuracy of diagnosis.

- Risk Stratification: mpMRI helps in risk stratification by characterizing the aggressiveness and extent of prostate cancer, aiding in treatment decision-making.

- Reduced Overdiagnosis: By guiding targeted biopsies, mpMRI reduces the likelihood of overdiagnosis and overtreatment of indolent prostate cancers.

Limitations of mpMRI:

- Cost: mpMRI can be expensive and may not be readily available in all healthcare settings.

- Operator Dependency: The quality and interpretation of mpMRI can vary depending on the experience of the radiologist.

- False Positives and Negatives: While highly accurate, mpMRI can yield false-positive or false-negative results in some cases.

2. Prostate-Specific Membrane Antigen (PSMA) PET/CT Imaging

Prostate-Specific Membrane Antigen (PSMA) positron emission tomography/computed tomography (PET/CT) imaging is an emerging advanced diagnostic technique that has gained prominence in the assessment of prostate cancer. PSMA is a protein that is overexpressed on the surface of prostate cancer cells. PSMA PET/CT imaging uses a radiolabeled molecule that binds to PSMA, allowing for the visualization of prostate cancer lesions with high precision.

Advantages of PSMA PET/CT Imaging:

- High Sensitivity: PSMA PET/CT imaging is highly sensitive in detecting both primary and metastatic prostate cancer lesions.

- Precise Localization: It provides precise localization of cancer lesions, helping in treatment planning and decision-making.

- Early Detection of Recurrence: PSMA PET/CT is valuable for detecting early biochemical recurrence after primary treatment, aiding in timely salvage therapies.

- Personalized Treatment: By accurately characterizing the extent and location of disease, PSMA PET/CT enables personalized treatment strategies.

Limitations of PSMA PET/CT Imaging:

- Availability: PSMA PET/CT imaging may not be widely available in all healthcare settings.

- Radiation Exposure: It involves exposure to ionizing radiation, which may limit its use in some cases.

- Cost: The cost of PSMA PET/CT imaging can be a barrier to access for some patients.

3. Liquid Biopsies

Liquid biopsies represent a non-invasive and promising approach to diagnosing and monitoring prostate cancer. These tests analyze various components in blood, urine, or other bodily fluids to detect genetic mutations, biomarkers, or circulating tumor cells associated with cancer. Key components of liquid biopsies for prostate cancer include:

- Circulating Tumor DNA (ctDNA): ctDNA refers to small fragments of DNA released into the bloodstream by cancer cells. Liquid biopsy tests can detect specific mutations in ctDNA that are associated with prostate cancer.

- Prostate Cancer Antigen 3 (PCA3) Test: The PCA3 test analyzes urine for the presence of PCA3 mRNA, a biomarker that is often elevated in prostate cancer.

- ExoDx Prostate (IntelliScore) Test: This urine-based test measures RNA expression levels to assess the risk of high-grade prostate cancer.

Advantages of Liquid Biopsies:

- Non-Invasive: Liquid biopsies are non-invasive and do not require tissue samples, reducing patient discomfort and risk.

- Monitoring: Liquid biopsies can be used for monitoring treatment response and disease progression.

- Personalized Treatment: They provide molecular information that can guide personalized treatment decisions.

Limitations of Liquid Biopsies:

- Sensitivity: Liquid biopsies may not detect all cases of prostate cancer, particularly in early stages.

- Specificity: False-positive results can occur, leading to unnecessary further testing or anxiety.

- Validation: The clinical utility and accuracy of liquid biopsy tests are still being validated in larger studies.

4. Prostate Fusion Biopsy

Prostate fusion biopsy, also known as targeted biopsy, is an advanced technique that combines imaging data, such as mpMRI, with real-time ultrasound to guide the biopsy needle to suspicious areas within the prostate gland. This approach allows for more precise sampling of suspicious lesions, reducing the risk of missing clinically significant prostate cancer.

Advantages of Prostate Fusion Biopsy:

- Precision: It precisely targets suspicious areas identified on imaging, improving the accuracy of diagnosis.

- Reduced Overdiagnosis: By focusing on suspicious lesions, fusion biopsy can reduce the likelihood of overdiagnosis of indolent prostate cancers.

- Treatment Guidance: Fusion biopsy provides valuable information for treatment planning and decision-making.

Limitations of Prostate Fusion Biopsy:

- Operator Skill: The accuracy of fusion biopsy depends on the experience and skill of the operator.

- Cost: The cost of fusion biopsy may be higher than that of conventional biopsies.

- Availability: Fusion biopsy may not be readily available in all healthcare settings.

5. Genomic Profiling

Genomic profiling involves the analysis of a patient's DNA to identify genetic mutations and alterations associated with prostate cancer. This advanced diagnostic technique provides insights into the molecular characteristics of an individual's cancer, helping to guide treatment decisions. Common genomic profiling tests for prostate cancer include:

- Oncotype DX Genomic Prostate Score: This test measures the expression of specific genes in prostate cancer tissue to predict the risk of disease aggressiveness.

- Decipher Genomic Classifier: Decipher analyzes the expression of genes in prostate cancer tissue to provide information about the likelihood of disease progression and response to treatment.

Advantages of Genomic Profiling:

- Personalized Treatment: Genomic profiling helps tailor treatment plans to the molecular characteristics of the patient's cancer.

- Risk Assessment: It provides information about the risk of disease progression, aiding in decision-making for treatment intensity.

- Avoiding Overtreatment: Genomic profiling can help identify low-risk cancers that may not require aggressive treatment.

Limitations of Genomic Profiling:

- Cost: Genomic profiling tests can be expensive and may not be covered by all insurance plans.

- Tissue Requirement: Genomic profiling typically requires a tissue sample, which may not be available or feasible in all cases.

- Clinical Validation: While promising, the clinical utility of genomic profiling is still being validated in larger studies.

6. Artificial Intelligence (AI) and Machine Learning

Artificial intelligence and machine learning techniques have shown great promise in improving the accuracy and efficiency of prostate cancer diagnosis and risk assessment. AI algorithms can analyze medical images, such as mpMRI scans, to detect suspicious lesions, classify cancer aggressiveness, and assist in treatment planning.

Advantages of AI and Machine Learning:

Enhanced Accuracy: AI algorithms can analyze large datasets and identify patterns that may not be apparent to human observers, improving diagnostic accuracy.

Efficiency: AI can streamline the interpretation of medical images, reducing the time required for diagnosis and treatment planning.

Risk Prediction: AI models can predict the risk of disease progression and help guide treatment decisions.

Limitations of AI and Machine Learning:

Validation: AI algorithms require rigorous validation to ensure their accuracy and reliability in clinical practice.

Data Quality: The performance of AI models depends on the quality and diversity of the data used for training.

Clinical Integration: Integrating AI into clinical practice and ensuring its accessibility to healthcare providers can be challenging.

Advanced diagnostic techniques have transformed the landscape of prostate cancer assessment, offering greater accuracy, precision, and personalization in diagnosis and treatment planning. While traditional methods such as PSA testing and DRE remain important, these advanced techniques, including mpMRI, PSMA PET/CT imaging, liquid biopsies, fusion biopsy, genomic profiling, and AI-driven approaches, have significantly enhanced our ability to detect and characterize prostate cancer.

The role of these advanced techniques extends beyond diagnosis; they also play a vital role in risk assessment, treatment selection, monitoring, and the avoidance of overdiagnosis and overtreatment. As research and technology continue to advance, the integration of these tools into clinical practice will further improve the management of prostate cancer, ultimately benefiting the well-being and outcomes of men affected by this disease. It is crucial for healthcare providers and patients to stay informed about these advancements and collaborate in making informed decisions regarding prostate cancer diagnosis and treatment.

CHAPTER TWO

Diet and Nutrition for Managing Prostate Cancer: A Comprehensive Guide

In this comprehensive guide, we will explore the impact of diet and nutrition on prostate cancer, including the foods to include and avoid, dietary patterns, supplements, and lifestyle choices that can support prostate health.

While certain risk factors, such as age and genetics, are beyond an individual's control, lifestyle factors, including diet and nutrition, can be modified to potentially reduce the risk of developing prostate cancer and improve outcomes for those diagnosed with the disease.

A growing body of research suggests that specific dietary choices and nutritional patterns may influence the development and progression of prostate cancer. It is essential to emphasize that while diet and nutrition can play a supportive role in prostate cancer management, they should not replace conventional medical treatments prescribed by healthcare professionals. Instead, diet and nutrition should be viewed as complementary strategies to enhance overall health and well-being during prostate cancer diagnosis, treatment, and survivorship.

Dietary Components for Prostate Health

Various dietary components have been studied for their potential impact on prostate health. These include:

1. Antioxidants

Antioxidants are compounds that help protect cells from oxidative damage caused by free radicals. Free radicals can damage DNA and are associated with cancer development. Common antioxidants include vitamins C and E, selenium, and beta-carotene.

2. Omega-3 Fatty Acids

Omega-3 fatty acids, found in fatty fish, flaxseeds, and walnuts, have anti-inflammatory properties that may help reduce inflammation, which is linked to cancer development.

3. Lycopene

Lycopene is a powerful antioxidant found in tomatoes, watermelon, and pink grapefruit. Some studies have suggested that lycopene-rich foods may lower the risk of prostate cancer.

4. Cruciferous Vegetables

Cruciferous vegetables, such as broccoli, cauliflower, and Brussels sprouts, contain compounds called glucosinolates, which may have anti-cancer properties.

5. Soy

Soy products contain phytoestrogens, which are plant-based compounds that can mimic estrogen in the body. Some studies have explored the potential benefits of soy in reducing the risk of prostate cancer, although the evidence is mixed.

6. Green Tea

Green tea contains polyphenols, which have antioxidant and anti-inflammatory properties. Some research has suggested that green tea consumption may be associated with a reduced risk of prostate cancer.

7. Vitamin D

Vitamin D is essential for bone health and may have a role in prostate cancer prevention and management. Adequate sun exposure and dietary sources of vitamin D, such as fortified dairy products and fatty fish, can help maintain healthy vitamin D levels.

Dietary Patterns for Prostate Health

In addition to individual dietary components, certain dietary patterns have been associated with prostate health:

1. Mediterranean Diet

The Mediterranean diet is characterized by a high intake of fruits, vegetables, whole grains, legumes, and olive oil, along with moderate consumption of fish, poultry, and red wine. This dietary pattern is rich in antioxidants, healthy fats, and fiber, making it a potentially beneficial choice for prostate health.

2. Plant-Based Diet

Plant-based diets, which emphasize fruits, vegetables, whole grains, nuts, seeds, and legumes while minimizing or excluding animal products, have been associated with a lower risk of various chronic diseases, including prostate cancer. These diets are typically high in fiber, antioxidants, and phytochemicals.

3. Low-Fat Diet

Some research has explored the potential benefits of a low-fat diet in prostate cancer management. Reducing dietary fat intake, particularly saturated fats, may be associated with improved outcomes for certain prostate cancer patients.

Foods to Include in a Prostate-Healthy Diet

Building a prostate-healthy diet involves incorporating a variety of foods that offer the nutrients and compounds associated with reduced cancer risk and improved prostate health. Here are some foods to include:

1. Fruits and Vegetables

Aim to consume a colorful array of fruits and vegetables, as different types offer various vitamins, minerals, and antioxidants. Berries, citrus fruits, leafy greens, tomatoes, and cruciferous vegetables are particularly beneficial.

2. Fatty Fish

Fatty fish like salmon, mackerel, and trout are rich in omega-3 fatty acids, which have anti-inflammatory properties. These fish also provide high-quality protein.

3. Nuts and Seeds

Almonds, walnuts, flaxseeds, and chia seeds are excellent sources of healthy fats, fiber, and antioxidants. They can be added to salads, yogurt, or enjoyed as snacks.

4. Legumes

Beans, lentils, and peas are rich in fiber and plant-based protein. They can be included in soups, stews, salads, and as side dishes.

5. Whole Grains

Choose whole grains like brown rice, quinoa, whole wheat pasta, and oats over refined grains. Whole grains are a source of fiber and provide sustained energy.

6. Herbs and Spices

Turmeric, ginger, garlic, and rosemary are examples of herbs and spices that have anti-inflammatory and antioxidant properties. They can be used to season dishes and add flavor.

7. Green Tea

Green tea contains polyphenols, particularly epigallocatechin gallate (EGCG), which may have anti-cancer properties. Enjoy a cup of green tea as part of your daily routine.

8. Lean Protein

Opt for lean protein sources such as skinless poultry, tofu, tempeh, and low-fat dairy products. These options provide essential nutrients without excessive saturated fat.

Foods to Limit or Avoid

While some foods and dietary patterns can support prostate health, others may have the opposite effect. Here are foods to limit or avoid:

1. Red and Processed Meats

High consumption of red and processed meats, such as beef, pork, and processed sausages, has been associated with an increased risk of prostate cancer. If you choose to consume red meat, opt for lean cuts and moderate portion sizes.

2. High-Fat Dairy Products

Full-fat dairy products, including whole milk and cheese, are sources of saturated fat. Consider lower-fat dairy options or dairy alternatives like almond milk or soy milk.

3. Excessive Sugar

A diet high in added sugars can contribute to obesity and inflammation, both of which are risk factors for cancer. Limit sugary beverages, sweets, and processed snacks.

4. Excessive Alcohol

Excessive alcohol consumption has been linked to an increased risk of various cancers, including prostate cancer. If you choose to drink alcohol, do so in moderation.

5. Trans Fats

Trans fats, often found in processed and fried foods, can promote inflammation and should be minimized in the diet.

Lifestyle Factors for Prostate Health

In addition to dietary choices, certain lifestyle factors can support prostate health:

1. Maintain a Healthy Weight

Obesity is associated with an increased risk of prostate cancer and more aggressive forms of the disease. Achieving and maintaining a healthy weight through diet and regular physical activity can reduce this risk.

2. Stay Physically Active

Regular physical activity, such as brisk walking, swimming, or cycling, is associated with a lower risk of prostate cancer and better outcomes for those diagnosed with the disease. Aim for at least 150 minutes of moderate-intensity exercise per week.

3. Manage Stress

Chronic stress can have a negative impact on overall health. Practices such as mindfulness, meditation, yoga, and deep breathing exercises can help manage stress.

4. Stay Hydrated

Adequate hydration is essential for overall health. Aim to drink plenty of water throughout the day.

5. Get Regular Check-Ups

Regular medical check-ups and cancer screenings are crucial for early detection and intervention. Discuss prostate cancer screening with your healthcare provider, especially if you have risk factors.

Supplements and Prostate Health

While a well-balanced diet is the preferred way to obtain nutrients, some individuals may consider dietary supplements to support prostate health. It is important to consult with a healthcare provider before taking supplements, as excessive or inappropriate use can have adverse effects. Common supplements for prostate health include:

1. Vitamin D

Vitamin D supplements may be recommended for individuals with low blood levels of vitamin D. Adequate vitamin D is important for bone health and overall well-being.

2. Selenium

Selenium is a trace mineral that plays a role in antioxidant defense. It is found in varying amounts in different foods and is also available as a supplement.

3. Omega-3 Fatty Acids

Omega-3 supplements, such as fish oil capsules, can provide the anti-inflammatory benefits of omega-3s. These supplements are often recommended for individuals who do not regularly consume fatty fish.

4. Saw Palmetto

Saw palmetto is an herbal supplement that some men take to alleviate urinary symptoms associated with benign prostatic hyperplasia (BPH), a non-cancerous enlargement of the prostate. Its effectiveness is a subject of debate, and it should be used under the guidance of a healthcare provider.

5. Lycopene

Lycopene supplements are available, but it is generally recommended to obtain lycopene from dietary sources like tomatoes and watermelon.

Diet and nutrition play a significant role in prostate health, offering the potential to reduce the risk of developing prostate cancer and improve outcomes for those diagnosed with the disease. A prostate-healthy diet is characterized by the inclusion of antioxidant-rich fruits and vegetables, omega-3 fatty acids, lycopene, cruciferous vegetables, soy, green tea, and vitamin D, along with limiting or avoiding red and processed meats, high-fat dairy products, excessive sugar, and alcohol.

Lifestyle factors, including maintaining a healthy weight, staying physically active, managing stress, and staying hydrated, also contribute to overall prostate health. Additionally, dietary supplements may be considered under the guidance of a healthcare provider, especially for individuals with specific nutritional deficiencies.

It is essential to approach dietary and lifestyle changes as part of a holistic approach to prostate cancer prevention and management. These changes should complement conventional medical treatments and be personalized to an individual's unique health profile and preferences. Regular consultation with a healthcare provider and a registered dietitian can provide guidance on making informed dietary and lifestyle choices to support prostate health and overall well-being.

Exercise and Physical Activity for Prostate Cancer

Prostate cancer is a significant health concern for men worldwide, and its management often involves a combination of medical treatments, lifestyle changes, and supportive interventions. Among these, exercise and physical activity have emerged as essential components in the prevention, treatment, and overall well-being of individuals with prostate cancer. In this comprehensive guide, we will explore the role of exercise and physical activity in prostate cancer, including their impact on prevention, treatment side effects, and overall quality of life.

While medical treatments such as surgery, radiation therapy, chemotherapy, and hormone therapy are essential in managing prostate cancer, emerging evidence highlights the critical role of lifestyle factors, including exercise and physical activity, in supporting prostate health.

Exercise and physical activity encompass a wide range of activities, from walking and swimming to strength training and yoga. These activities offer numerous physical and psychological benefits that can significantly impact the prevention, treatment, and recovery from prostate cancer. It is important to note that exercise should be tailored to an individual's fitness level and health status, and consultation with a healthcare provider is recommended before starting or significantly changing an exercise routine.

Benefits of Exercise and Physical Activity for Prostate Cancer

Exercise and physical activity offer a multitude of benefits for individuals at risk of or diagnosed with prostate cancer. These benefits extend to both physical and emotional well-being:

1. Reducing Prostate Cancer Risk

Emerging research suggests that regular physical activity may lower the risk of developing prostate cancer. Exercise can help regulate hormones, reduce inflammation, and support a healthy body weight, all of which are factors associated with reduced cancer risk.

2. Improving Treatment Tolerance

For individuals undergoing prostate cancer treatment, such as surgery, radiation therapy, or chemotherapy, exercise can enhance treatment tolerance and recovery. It can help maintain muscle mass, reduce fatigue, and improve overall physical functioning during and after treatment.

3. Managing Treatment Side Effects

Exercise has been shown to effectively manage treatment-related side effects common in prostate cancer, including fatigue, urinary incontinence, and sexual dysfunction. It can also aid in maintaining bone health, which is particularly important for individuals undergoing hormone therapy that can lead to bone loss.

4. Enhancing Quality of Life

Regular physical activity can have a profound impact on the overall quality of life for prostate cancer survivors. Exercise can boost mood, reduce anxiety and depression, improve sleep, and enhance self-esteem, helping individuals cope with the emotional and psychological challenges that often accompany a cancer diagnosis.

5. Promoting Cardiovascular Health

Many prostate cancer treatments, including hormone therapy, can increase the risk of cardiovascular issues. Exercise plays a crucial role in promoting cardiovascular health, reducing the risk of heart disease, and mitigating the cardiovascular side effects of treatment.

6. Supporting Bone Health

Prostate cancer treatment can sometimes lead to reduced bone density and an increased risk of fractures. Weight-bearing exercises, such as walking or weightlifting, can help support bone health and reduce this risk.

7. Enhancing Immune Function

Regular physical activity has been shown to strengthen the immune system, potentially aiding the body's ability to fight cancer cells and infections.

8. Building Resilience

Engaging in regular exercise can instill a sense of empowerment and resilience, helping individuals feel more in control of their health and cancer journey.

Types of Exercise and Physical Activity

Exercise and physical activity encompass various types, each offering unique benefits. A well-rounded exercise routine may include:

1. Aerobic Exercise

Aerobic exercises, such as walking, jogging, swimming, and cycling, elevate the heart rate and improve cardiovascular fitness. These activities can help with weight management, reduce fatigue, and enhance overall endurance.

2. Strength Training

Strength training exercises, which involve resistance or weight-bearing activities, help build and maintain muscle mass. These exercises can be particularly beneficial for countering muscle loss that may occur during cancer treatment.

3. Flexibility and Stretching

Flexibility and stretching exercises, such as yoga and Pilates, improve joint mobility and muscle flexibility. They can help reduce muscle tension, improve posture, and enhance overall comfort.

4. Balance and Coordination

Balance and coordination exercises, which may include tai chi or specific balance drills, can help reduce the risk of falls and improve stability, which is essential for individuals with bone health concerns.

5. Pelvic Floor Exercises

Pelvic floor exercises, such as Kegel exercises, can aid in managing urinary incontinence, a common side effect of prostate cancer treatment.

6. Relaxation Techniques

Mind-body practices like meditation and deep breathing exercises can reduce stress, anxiety, and depression, improving overall mental well-being.

Exercise Guidelines for Prostate Cancer

While the benefits of exercise for prostate cancer are clear, it is important to approach physical activity with care and consideration of an individual's unique health status and treatment plan. Here are some general guidelines:

1. Consult with a Healthcare Provider

Before beginning or significantly changing an exercise routine, it is essential to consult with a healthcare provider, particularly if you are currently undergoing treatment or have specific health concerns. Your healthcare provider can offer personalized recommendations and address any potential exercise-related risks.

2. Start Slowly

For individuals who are new to exercise or have been sedentary for a while, it is advisable to start slowly and gradually increase the intensity and duration of physical activity. This approach reduces the risk of injury and allows the body to adapt.

3. Tailor Exercise to Individual Needs

Exercise should be tailored to an individual's fitness level, physical abilities, and treatment-related side effects. Some individuals may need to modify exercises or engage in specific rehabilitation programs.

4. Aim for Regularity

Consistency is key when it comes to exercise. Aim for regular physical activity, incorporating a variety of exercises to address different aspects of fitness, including cardiovascular fitness, strength, flexibility, and balance.

5. Listen to Your Body

It is important to listen to your body and be aware of any discomfort or pain during exercise. If you experience pain or discomfort, it is advisable to stop the activity and consult with your healthcare provider.

6. Hydration and Nutrition

Proper hydration and nutrition are essential to support physical activity. Staying well-hydrated and consuming a balanced diet with adequate nutrients is crucial for energy and recovery.

7. Consider Professional Guidance

Working with a certified fitness trainer or physical therapist with experience in cancer care can provide valuable guidance and support in developing a safe and effective exercise program.

8. Set Realistic Goals

Set achievable goals based on your current fitness level and treatment status. Celebrate your progress, no matter how small, and be patient with yourself.

Exercise and Specific Treatment Modalities

The role of exercise may vary depending on the specific treatment modalities used for prostate cancer:

1. Surgery

For individuals undergoing prostatectomy (surgery to remove the prostate), exercise can help with preoperative conditioning, postoperative recovery, and reducing the risk of postoperative complications, such as blood clots and urinary incontinence. Post-surgery, it is essential to follow surgical guidelines and gradually reintroduce exercise under the guidance of healthcare providers.

2. Radiation Therapy

Radiation therapy can cause fatigue and changes in muscle and bone density. Engaging in regular exercise, particularly strength training and weight-bearing activities, can help maintain muscle and bone health. It is important to consult with radiation oncologists and exercise specialists to tailor an exercise plan to individual needs.

3. Hormone Therapy

Hormone therapy may lead to muscle loss, weight gain, and reduced bone density. Exercise, including strength training and weight-bearing activities, can mitigate these side effects and promote overall well-being.

4. Chemotherapy

Chemotherapy can cause fatigue and muscle weakness. Exercise can help counter these effects, improve energy levels, and support overall functioning. It is essential to discuss exercise plans with oncologists to ensure compatibility with chemotherapy regimens.

Exercise and physical activity play a crucial role in prostate cancer prevention, treatment, and overall well-being. Regular physical activity can reduce cancer risk, enhance treatment tolerance, manage treatment side effects, improve quality of life, and promote physical and mental health.

Individuals at risk of or diagnosed with prostate cancer should approach exercise with guidance from healthcare providers, taking into account their specific health status and treatment plan. Exercise programs should be tailored to individual needs, gradually increasing in intensity and duration, and encompassing various types of activities to address different aspects of fitness.

Exercise is not a replacement for medical treatment but should be viewed as a complementary and supportive strategy to optimize prostate cancer management and overall health. Engaging in regular physical activity can empower individuals on their cancer journey, improve their sense of well-being, and contribute to a healthier, more active lifestyle during and beyond prostate cancer treatment.

Stress Management in Prostate Cancer

A diagnosis of prostate cancer is a life-altering event that can trigger a range of emotional and psychological responses. The journey from diagnosis through treatment and recovery is often marked by uncertainty, fear, and stress. Stress, in particular, can have profound effects on both the physical and emotional well-being of individuals with prostate cancer. However, effective stress management strategies can help individuals navigate the challenges of prostate cancer, improve their quality of life, and foster a sense of resilience. In this discussion, we will explore the impact of stress on prostate cancer, the factors contributing to stress, and practical stress management techniques for individuals on this journey.

Understanding Stress in the Context of Prostate Cancer

Stress is a natural response to life's challenges and uncertainties. In the context of prostate cancer, stress can manifest in various ways, affecting an individual's emotional, psychological, and physical well-being. Some common stressors for individuals with prostate cancer include:

1. Diagnosis Shock and Uncertainty: The moment of diagnosis can be overwhelming, often leading to a state of shock and disbelief. Uncertainty about the disease's progression, treatment outcomes, and future can intensify stress.

2. Treatment Decisions: Deciding on a treatment plan can be a complex and anxiety-inducing process. Questions about the potential side effects, risks, and benefits of various treatment options can lead to heightened stress.

3. Treatment Side Effects: The physical and emotional toll of prostate cancer treatments, such as surgery, radiation therapy, and hormone therapy, can contribute to stress. Side effects like fatigue, pain, incontinence, and sexual dysfunction can impact quality of life.

4. Fear of Recurrence: Even after successful treatment, the fear of cancer recurrence can linger. This fear can manifest as ongoing stress and anxiety.

5. Lifestyle Changes: Prostate cancer and its treatments may necessitate significant lifestyle changes, including dietary modifications, exercise routines, and stress management practices. Adjusting to these changes can be challenging and stressful.

6. Impact on Relationships: Prostate cancer can affect relationships with partners, family members, and friends. Communication difficulties, role changes, and emotional strain can generate stress within interpersonal relationships.

7. Financial Concerns: The cost of prostate cancer treatment, coupled with potential work-related disruptions, can create financial stress for individuals and their families.

8. Emotional and Psychological Well-Being: The emotional toll of prostate cancer, including anxiety, depression, and feelings of isolation, can contribute to overall stress levels.

It is important to recognize that stress is a normal reaction to these challenges and that individuals with prostate cancer are not alone in experiencing it. Acknowledging and addressing stress can lead to improved emotional and physical well-being and enhance one's ability to cope with the demands of prostate cancer.

The Impact of Stress on Prostate Cancer

Stress can have a profound impact on both the mind and body, affecting individuals with prostate cancer in several ways:

1. Physical Health: Chronic stress can weaken the immune system, making the body more susceptible to infections and illnesses. For individuals with prostate cancer, a compromised immune system may hinder the body's ability to fight cancer cells effectively.

2. Treatment Tolerance: Stress can exacerbate treatment-related side effects, such as fatigue, pain, and nausea, making it more challenging for individuals to tolerate and adhere to their treatment regimens.

3. Emotional Well-Being: Prolonged stress can lead to anxiety, depression, and a diminished sense of well-being. These emotional challenges can hinder one's ability to cope with prostate cancer and make informed treatment decisions.

4. Sleep Disturbances: Stress often disrupts sleep patterns, leading to insomnia or poor-quality sleep. Adequate rest is essential for physical and emotional recovery, making sleep disturbances a significant concern for individuals with prostate cancer.

5. Coping Mechanisms: Individuals under stress may resort to unhealthy coping mechanisms, such as excessive alcohol consumption or tobacco use, which can negatively impact overall health.

Practical Stress Management Techniques

Effectively managing stress is essential for individuals with prostate cancer to enhance their overall well-being and improve their ability to navigate the challenges of the disease. Here are practical stress management techniques to consider:

1. Seek Support

- Healthcare Providers: Open and honest communication with healthcare providers can provide valuable information about the disease, treatment options, and expectations, reducing uncertainty and anxiety.

- Support Groups: Joining prostate cancer support groups or online communities can connect individuals with others facing similar challenges. Sharing experiences and receiving support from peers can be reassuring and reduce feelings of isolation.

- Mental Health Professionals: Consultation with a therapist, counselor, or psychologist can provide tools and strategies to manage stress, anxiety, and depression effectively.

2. Maintain Open Communication

- Family and Friends: Engage in open and honest conversations with loved ones about the impact of prostate cancer on your life and relationships. Effective communication can foster understanding and support.

- Partners: For individuals in romantic relationships, maintaining open communication with partners about intimacy, sexual health, and emotional needs is crucial.

3. Practice Relaxation Techniques

- Mindfulness Meditation: Mindfulness practices, such as meditation and deep breathing exercises, can reduce stress, improve emotional well-being, and enhance overall resilience.

- Progressive Muscle Relaxation: This technique involves tensing and then relaxing various muscle groups in the body, promoting physical relaxation and stress reduction.

4. Physical Activity

- Regular Exercise: Engaging in regular physical activity, such as walking, swimming, or yoga, can boost mood, reduce stress, and improve overall well-being. Exercise is also associated with improved treatment tolerance and reduced fatigue.

5. Maintain a Healthy Lifestyle

- Diet: A balanced diet that includes a variety of nutrient-rich foods can support overall health and well-being. Consider consulting with a registered dietitian for personalized dietary guidance.

- Sleep: Prioritize good sleep hygiene practices to improve sleep quality and duration. This may include establishing a bedtime routine, creating a comfortable sleep environment, and avoiding caffeine and electronic devices before bedtime.

6. Set Realistic Goals

- Goal Setting: Establish realistic and achievable goals for managing stress and prostate cancer. Celebrate even small accomplishments and progress in your journey.

7. Limit Exposure to Stressors

- Information Overload: While it's essential to stay informed about prostate cancer and treatment options, limit exposure to excessive information and avoid constant internet searching, which can contribute to stress and anxiety.

8. Mind-Body Practices

- Yoga and Tai Chi: Mind-body practices like yoga and tai chi combine physical movement with mindfulness techniques, promoting relaxation, stress reduction, and improved flexibility.

9. Professional Support

- Therapy: Consider individual or group therapy to explore and address stressors, emotional challenges, and coping strategies.

10. Self-Care

- Time for Yourself: Make time for activities you enjoy, hobbies, and self-care practices that nurture your overall well-being.

Managing stress is an integral part of the journey for individuals with prostate cancer. While the emotional and psychological challenges of the disease are undeniable, effective stress management strategies can help individuals navigate these challenges with resilience and well-being. Seeking support, maintaining open communication, practicing relaxation techniques, engaging in physical activity, and adopting a healthy lifestyle can significantly reduce stress and enhance overall quality of life.

It is essential for individuals with prostate cancer to recognize that they are not alone in their experience of stress and that seeking help and support is a sign of strength, not weakness. By embracing stress management techniques and building a support network, individuals with prostate cancer can nurture their well-being and face the challenges of their journey with greater resilience and optimism.

CHAPTER THREE

Herbal Remedies and Supplements in Prostate Cancer

While medical treatments such as surgery, radiation therapy, and hormone therapy are established approaches to managing prostate cancer, interest in complementary and alternative therapies, including herbal remedies and supplements, has been on the rise. This interest stems from the desire to explore additional treatment options, alleviate treatment-related side effects, and improve overall well-being. In this comprehensive discussion, we will examine the role of herbal remedies and supplements in prostate cancer, the evidence supporting their use, and the important considerations individuals should be aware of when incorporating these therapies into their prostate cancer management.

Each treatment approach is carefully selected based on the individual's cancer stage, risk factors, and overall health. While conventional medical treatments have shown efficacy in managing prostate cancer, some individuals explore complementary and alternative therapies to complement their treatment plans or alleviate treatment-related side effects.

Herbal remedies and dietary supplements have gained popularity among individuals with prostate cancer due to their perceived natural and holistic nature. However, it is essential to approach these therapies with caution and under the guidance of healthcare providers, as they may interact with conventional treatments, have adverse effects, or lack substantial scientific evidence supporting their use.

Common Herbal Remedies and Supplements in Prostate Cancer

A wide range of herbal remedies and dietary supplements are often considered by individuals with prostate cancer. These include:

1. Saw Palmetto

Saw palmetto is derived from the fruit of the American dwarf palm tree and is commonly used to alleviate urinary symptoms associated with benign prostatic hyperplasia (BPH). Some individuals with prostate cancer turn to saw palmetto to manage urinary issues, but its effectiveness in this context remains a subject of debate.

2. Green Tea

Green tea is rich in polyphenols, particularly epigallocatechin gallate (EGCG), which have antioxidant and anti-inflammatory properties. Some studies have explored the potential benefits of green tea in reducing the risk of prostate cancer or inhibiting its progression, although the evidence is inconclusive.

3. Pomegranate

Pomegranate and pomegranate extract have garnered attention for their potential anti-cancer properties. Some research suggests that pomegranate may slow the progression of prostate cancer or reduce treatment-related side effects, but more extensive studies are needed to establish its efficacy.

4. Turmeric/Curcumin

Turmeric, a spice commonly used in Indian cuisine, contains curcumin, a compound with anti-inflammatory and antioxidant properties. Some studies have investigated curcumin's potential role in inhibiting prostate cancer growth, but the clinical evidence remains limited.

5. Vitamin D

Vitamin D is essential for bone health and overall well-being. Adequate vitamin D levels may be important for individuals with prostate cancer, particularly those undergoing hormone therapy that can affect bone density.

6. Selenium

Selenium is a trace mineral that plays a role in antioxidant defense. Some studies have explored selenium's potential in reducing the risk of prostate cancer, but the results have been mixed, and excessive selenium intake can have adverse effects.

7. Zinc

Zinc is a mineral that supports various bodily functions, including immune function and wound healing. Some research has investigated the relationship between zinc levels and prostate cancer risk, but the findings are inconclusive.

8. Omega-3 Fatty Acids

Omega-3 fatty acids, found in fatty fish, flaxseeds, and walnuts, have anti-inflammatory properties and may be associated with a reduced risk of prostate cancer progression or improved treatment tolerance.

9. Essiac Tea

Essiac tea is a herbal tea blend that includes burdock root, slippery elm bark, sheep sorrel, and Indian rhubarb root. It has been promoted as a natural cancer remedy, including for prostate cancer, but there is no scientific evidence to support its effectiveness.

10. Modified Citrus Pectin

Modified citrus pectin is a dietary fiber derived from citrus fruits. Some studies have suggested that it may have potential in inhibiting prostate cancer metastasis, but further research is needed to confirm these findings.

The Evidence and Considerations

When considering the use of herbal remedies and supplements in prostate cancer, it is crucial to weigh the available evidence and take several factors into account:

1. Lack of Standardization

Herbal remedies and dietary supplements are not standardized like pharmaceutical drugs. The composition, purity, and potency of these products can vary widely among brands and formulations, making it challenging to establish consistent therapeutic effects.

2. Limited Scientific Evidence

Many herbal remedies and supplements lack robust scientific evidence to support their efficacy in preventing, treating, or managing prostate cancer. While some studies suggest potential benefits, larger and more rigorous clinical trials are needed to confirm these findings.

3. Potential Interactions

Herbal remedies and supplements can interact with conventional prostate cancer treatments, affecting their effectiveness or causing adverse effects. It is crucial for individuals to inform their healthcare providers about any supplements they are taking to prevent potential interactions.

4. Safety Concerns

Some herbal remedies and supplements may have adverse effects, particularly when taken in excessive amounts. For example, high doses of certain vitamins and minerals can lead to toxicity.

5. Delay or Discontinuation of Conventional Treatment

Relying solely on herbal remedies and supplements as a substitute for conventional medical treatments can delay or jeopardize the effectiveness of established treatments, potentially allowing cancer to progress.

6. Personalized Approach

Prostate cancer is a highly individualized disease, and what works for one person may not work for another. Treatment decisions, including the use of herbal remedies and supplements, should be personalized and made in consultation with healthcare providers.

7. Monitoring and Evaluation

Individuals who choose to incorporate herbal remedies and supplements into their prostate cancer management should undergo regular monitoring and evaluation to assess treatment response, side effects, and overall well-being.

8. Consultation with Healthcare Providers

Individuals should always consult with their healthcare providers before starting any herbal remedies or supplements, especially when undergoing conventional prostate cancer treatments. Healthcare providers can offer guidance on potential interactions, dosages, and monitoring.

Herbal remedies and supplements have gained popularity among individuals with prostate cancer as complementary and alternative therapies. While some of these therapies may hold promise, it is crucial to approach them with caution and an understanding of their limitations. The evidence supporting the use of herbal remedies and supplements in prostate cancer is often limited and inconclusive, and their safety and efficacy can vary widely.

Individuals with prostate cancer should prioritize open communication with their healthcare providers, engage in shared decision-making regarding treatment options, and consider a holistic approach that encompasses conventional medical treatments, lifestyle modifications, and supportive therapies. Ultimately, the goal is to optimize the overall well-being and quality of life of individuals with prostate cancer while prioritizing safe and evidence-based approaches to treatment and management.

Alternative Therapies in Prostate Cancer

In this comprehensive discussion, we will explore alternative therapies in prostate cancer, their potential benefits, the evidence supporting their use, and the critical considerations individuals should keep in mind when considering these approaches.

While conventional medical treatments remain the primary approach to prostate cancer, there is growing interest in complementary and alternative therapies to enhance treatment outcomes, alleviate side effects, and promote overall well-being.

Alternative therapies encompass a wide range of practices, including dietary supplements, mind-body techniques, physical therapies, and energy-based approaches. It is important to note that alternative therapies should not replace established medical treatments for prostate cancer but can be used as adjuncts to address specific needs and preferences.

Common Alternative Therapies in Prostate Cancer

Numerous alternative therapies are considered by individuals with prostate cancer. These include:

1. Acupuncture

Acupuncture involves the insertion of thin needles into specific points on the body to promote energy flow and balance. Some individuals with prostate cancer use acupuncture to alleviate treatment-related side effects, such as pain, nausea, and fatigue.

2. Yoga and Tai Chi

Mind-body practices like yoga and tai chi combine physical movement with mindfulness techniques, promoting relaxation, stress reduction, and improved flexibility. They can help individuals with prostate cancer manage stress, improve physical functioning, and enhance overall well-being.

3. Massage Therapy

Massage therapy involves the manipulation of muscles and soft tissues to reduce tension, relieve pain, and promote relaxation. It can be particularly beneficial for individuals experiencing muscle pain or tension as a result of treatment.

4. Mindfulness-Based Stress Reduction (MBSR)

MBSR is a structured program that teaches mindfulness meditation techniques to reduce stress and enhance overall well-being. It can be valuable for individuals with prostate cancer coping with stress, anxiety, or depression.

5. Dietary Supplements

Various dietary supplements, such as vitamins, minerals, herbal remedies, and antioxidants, are often considered by individuals with prostate cancer to support their overall health, boost the immune system, or alleviate specific treatment-related side effects.

6. Ayurvedic Medicine

Ayurveda is a traditional system of medicine from India that emphasizes holistic well-being through a combination of dietary recommendations, herbal remedies, and lifestyle practices. Some individuals with prostate cancer explore Ayurvedic approaches to promote balance and well-being.

7. Energy-Based Therapies

Energy-based therapies, such as Reiki and healing touch, involve the manipulation of energy fields to promote relaxation and healing. These therapies are sometimes used to reduce stress and enhance overall well-being.

8. Traditional Chinese Medicine (TCM)

TCM includes practices like acupuncture, herbal medicine, and qigong. Some individuals with prostate cancer explore TCM as a complementary approach to address specific symptoms or promote overall health.

The Evidence and Considerations

When considering alternative therapies in prostate cancer, it is essential to weigh the available evidence, potential benefits, and critical considerations:

1. Limited Scientific Evidence

Many alternative therapies lack robust scientific evidence to support their efficacy in treating or managing prostate cancer. While some studies suggest potential benefits, larger and more rigorous clinical trials are needed to confirm these findings.

2. Potential for Interaction

Alternative therapies can interact with conventional prostate cancer treatments, affecting their effectiveness or causing adverse effects. It is crucial for individuals to inform their healthcare providers about any alternative therapies they are considering to prevent potential interactions.

3. Safety Concerns

Some alternative therapies may have adverse effects, particularly when administered by untrained or unqualified practitioners. Ensuring that practitioners are licensed, certified, or experienced in their respective fields is essential.

4. Personalized Approach

Prostate cancer is a highly individualized disease, and what works for one person may not work for another. Treatment decisions, including the use of alternative therapies, should be personalized and made in consultation with healthcare providers.

5. Monitoring and Evaluation

Individuals who choose to incorporate alternative therapies into their prostate cancer management should undergo regular monitoring and evaluation to assess treatment response, side effects, and overall well-being.

6. Communication with Healthcare Providers

Open and transparent communication with healthcare providers is crucial when considering alternative therapies. Healthcare providers can offer guidance on potential interactions, safety concerns, and monitoring.

7. Shared Decision-Making

Treatment decisions should be made collaboratively between individuals with prostate cancer and their healthcare providers, taking into account the individual's cancer stage, risk factors, and overall health.

8. Avoiding Delay of Conventional Treatment

Relying solely on alternative therapies as a replacement for established medical treatments can delay or jeopardize the effectiveness of conventional treatments, potentially allowing cancer to progress.

9. Cost Considerations

Alternative therapies can vary widely in cost, and insurance coverage may not be available for these approaches. Individuals should consider the financial implications of alternative therapies and discuss them with their healthcare providers.

10. Psychological and Emotional Support

Alternative therapies can provide psychological and emotional support for individuals with prostate cancer, helping them cope with stress, anxiety, and depression. These therapies may complement conventional psychological support services.

Alternative therapies in prostate cancer are a subject of interest and exploration for many individuals seeking holistic approaches to complement their conventional treatments. While some alternative therapies may offer potential benefits in terms of symptom management, stress reduction, and overall well-being, it is essential to approach them with caution and awareness of their limitations.

The evidence supporting the use of alternative therapies in prostate cancer is often limited and inconclusive. Healthcare providers should prioritize open communication with their patients and engage in shared decision-making that considers individual cancer characteristics, treatment goals, and patient preferences.

Ultimately, the goal is to optimize the overall well-being and quality of life of individuals with prostate cancer while prioritizing safe and evidence-based approaches to treatment and management. By taking a personalized and integrated approach that encompasses conventional medical treatments, lifestyle modifications, and supportive therapies, individuals with prostate cancer can enhance their overall health and well-being on their journey toward prostate cancer management and recovery.

Mind-Body Practices for Managing Prostate Cancer

Emotions, stress, anxiety, and quality of life are vital aspects of the prostate cancer experience that can greatly benefit from holistic approaches. Mind-body practices, a category of complementary therapies, offer a holistic perspective on managing prostate cancer, focusing on the interconnectedness of the mind and body. In this comprehensive exploration, we will delve into the world of mind-body practices and their role in supporting the well-being of individuals with prostate cancer.

The journey from diagnosis through treatment and recovery can be physically and emotionally challenging, often impacting the mental and emotional aspects of an individual's life. Mind-body practices are a category of complementary therapies that recognize the profound connection between mental and physical health. These practices aim to promote overall well-being by fostering harmony between the mind, body, and spirit.

Mind-body practices encompass a wide range of techniques and approaches that have been studied for their potential benefits in managing prostate cancer. While they are not a replacement for medical treatment, mind-body practices can significantly enhance the quality of life, emotional well-being, and physical comfort of individuals with prostate cancer.

Understanding Mind-Body Practices

Mind-body practices are based on the principle that the mind and body are interconnected, and the state of one can influence the other. These practices recognize the power of the mind in promoting healing, reducing stress, and enhancing overall well-being. Some common mind-body practices Practice

1. Meditation

Meditation involves focused attention and mental discipline to cultivate mindfulness, relaxation, and inner peace. It can help individuals with prostate cancer manage stress, reduce anxiety, and improve their emotional well-being.

2. Yoga

Yoga combines physical postures, breathing exercises, and mindfulness techniques to promote flexibility, strength, and relaxation. It can enhance physical comfort, reduce muscle tension, and alleviate stress for individuals with prostate cancer.

3. Tai Chi

Tai Chi is a mind-body practice that involves slow, flowing movements and deep breathing. It improves balance, flexibility, and overall physical functioning, making it particularly beneficial for individuals with prostate cancer experiencing mobility challenges.

4. Progressive Muscle Relaxation (PMR)

PMR is a technique that involves systematically tensing and relaxing muscle groups to reduce tension, alleviate pain, and promote relaxation. It can be helpful for individuals with prostate cancer experiencing muscle discomfort.

5. Guided Imagery

Guided imagery is a practice where individuals use their imagination to create positive mental images, fostering relaxation and emotional well-being. It can be particularly useful in managing stress and anxiety.

6. Biofeedback

Biofeedback is a technique that allows individuals to monitor and control physiological responses, such as heart rate and muscle tension, to promote relaxation and stress reduction.

The Role of Mind-Body Practices in Prostate Cancer Management

Mind-body practices play a multifaceted role in prostate cancer management, addressing various aspects of the disease and its impact on individuals' lives:

1. Stress Reduction

Stress is a common emotional response to a prostate cancer diagnosis and the subsequent treatment journey. Chronic stress can have negative effects on physical health and overall well-being. Mind-body practices like meditation, yoga, and Tai Chi are effective tools for reducing stress levels. Regular practice can enhance an individual's ability to cope with the emotional challenges of prostate cancer.

2. Pain Management

Prostate cancer and its treatments may cause physical discomfort and pain. Mind-body practices, including progressive muscle relaxation and guided imagery, can be instrumental in alleviating pain and promoting physical comfort. These practices teach individuals how to relax tense muscles and manage pain more effectively.

3. Emotional Well-Being

Prostate cancer can elicit a range of emotions, including fear, anxiety, sadness, and anger. Mind-body practices provide a safe and supportive environment for individuals to explore and process these emotions. Guided imagery and meditation can help individuals cultivate emotional resilience and a more positive outlook.

4. Enhancing Quality of Life

Prostate cancer can impact various aspects of an individual's life, including relationships, sexual function, and overall quality of life. Mind-body practices can promote self-awareness, self-acceptance, and a sense of empowerment, helping individuals navigate these challenges more effectively.

5. Improved Physical Functioning

Physical activity is often recommended for individuals with prostate cancer to enhance overall physical functioning and reduce treatment-related side effects. Mind-body practices like yoga and Tai Chi offer a gentle and low-impact way to improve flexibility, balance, and strength, making them suitable for individuals with varying fitness levels.

6. Immune System Support

Chronic stress can weaken the immune system, potentially impacting the body's ability to fight cancer cells and infections. Mind-body practices that reduce stress and promote relaxation may support the immune system's function.

7. Coping with Treatment Side Effects

Prostate cancer treatments can lead to side effects like fatigue, urinary incontinence, and sexual dysfunction. Mind-body practices can help individuals manage these treatment-related challenges by enhancing physical comfort and emotional well-being.

8. Complementary to Medical Treatment

It is essential to emphasize that mind-body practices are not a replacement for medical treatment. Rather, they complement conventional medical approaches to prostate cancer management. These practices can enhance the overall well-being and quality of life of individuals with prostate cancer, helping them navigate the emotional and physical challenges of the disease.

Incorporating Mind-Body Practices into Prostate Cancer Management

Incorporating mind-body practices into prostate cancer management requires a thoughtful and individualized approach. Here are some steps individuals can consider:

1. Consultation with Healthcare Providers

Before starting any mind-body practice, individuals should consult with their healthcare providers, particularly if they have underlying medical conditions or specific health concerns. Healthcare providers can offer guidance on the safety and suitability of these practices.

2. Seek Qualified Instructors

When participating in mind-body practices like yoga or Tai Chi, individuals should seek qualified instructors who have experience working with individuals with cancer or chronic health conditions. Instructors should be knowledgeable about adaptations and modifications to accommodate physical limitations.

3. Establish a Consistent Practice

Consistency is key to reaping the benefits of mind-body practices. Individuals should establish a regular practice schedule, incorporating these techniques into their daily or weekly routines.

4. Mindful Self-Care

Mind-body practices encourage mindful self-care and self-compassion. Individuals should approach these practices with an open heart and a non-judgmental attitude, allowing themselves to explore their emotions and physical sensations.

5. Integrative Approach

Individuals should view mind-body practices as part of an integrative approach to prostate cancer management. These practices work in conjunction with medical treatments and other supportive interventions to enhance overall well-being.

6. Set Realistic Goals

Setting realistic goals for mind-body practices is essential. Individuals should focus on their own progress and well-being rather than comparing themselves to others or expecting immediate results.

7. Supportive Community

Participating in mind-body practices within a supportive community can enhance the experience and provide emotional support. Consider joining classes or groups specifically designed for individuals with cancer.

Mind-body practices offer a holistic approach to managing prostate cancer by recognizing the interconnectedness of the mind and body. These practices can have a profound impact on stress reduction, pain management, emotional well-being, and overall quality of life for individuals with prostate cancer.

It is important for individuals to approach mind-body practices with an open mind, seeking guidance from healthcare providers and qualified instructors. By incorporating these practices into their prostate cancer management plan, individuals can foster physical and emotional resilience, enhance their overall well-being, and navigate the challenges of prostate cancer with greater confidence and inner peace.

CHAPTER FOUR

Active Surveillance in Prostate Cancer

Active Surveillance is an approach that has gained prominence in recent years for managing low-risk prostate cancer, offering a prudent alternative to immediate intervention. In this comprehensive discussion, we will explore Active Surveillance as a strategy for prostate cancer management, examining its principles, eligibility criteria, benefits, and potential challenges.

Active Surveillance is an approach that has emerged as an effective and evidence-based strategy for managing low-risk prostate cancer. Rather than opting for immediate treatment, Active Surveillance involves a systematic monitoring and evaluation process to assess the progression of the disease over time. This approach aims to spare individuals from unnecessary treatment-related side effects while reserving intervention for cases where it is truly warranted.

Understanding Active Surveillance

Active Surveillance is rooted in the principle of "watchful waiting" but differs in its systematic and proactive approach to monitoring the disease. While watchful waiting may involve minimal intervention and a passive stance toward the disease's progression, Active Surveillance takes a more active role in tracking the cancer's behavior and progression.

Key components of Active Surveillance include:

1. Regular Monitoring: Individuals on Active Surveillance undergo regular check-ups and monitoring, which may include prostate-specific antigen (PSA) tests, digital rectal examinations (DRE), and periodic prostate biopsies. The frequency of these assessments is determined by the individual's risk profile and the clinician's recommendations.

2. Risk Assessment: Healthcare providers use various criteria to assess an individual's risk profile, including PSA levels, Gleason score (a measure of cancer aggressiveness based on biopsy results), and clinical stage. Low-risk prostate cancer is typically characterized by PSA levels below a certain threshold, low Gleason scores, and the absence of extensive disease involvement.

3. Biopsy Confirmation: The diagnosis of prostate cancer is confirmed through a prostate biopsy, which involves obtaining tissue samples from the prostate gland. The biopsy results help determine the cancer's grade and aggressiveness.

4. Shared Decision-Making: The decision to pursue Active Surveillance is made collaboratively between the individual and the healthcare provider. Factors such as age, overall health, preferences, and the potential risks and benefits of treatment are considered.

5. Regular Follow-up: Individuals on Active Surveillance are closely followed by a multidisciplinary healthcare team, which may include urologists, oncologists, and radiologists. These specialists work together to monitor the disease's progression and discuss treatment options if needed.

Eligibility Criteria for Active Surveillance

Active Surveillance is not suitable for all individuals with prostate cancer. It is typically recommended for those with low-risk disease, characterized by specific criteria, including:

1. Low PSA Levels: PSA levels below a certain threshold (usually 10 ng/mL or lower) are indicative of low-risk disease.

2. Low Gleason Score: A Gleason score of 6 or less on the biopsy indicates well-differentiated and less aggressive cancer cells.

3. Low Clinical Stage: Clinical staging (based on physical examination and imaging) reveals localized disease with no signs of spread beyond the prostate gland.

4. Negative Biopsy: The biopsy results should confirm the absence of extensive cancer involvement in multiple cores of the prostate.

5. Age and Health Status: Older individuals or those with significant comorbidities that may limit life expectancy may be candidates for Active Surveillance, as the potential benefits of aggressive treatment may be outweighed by the risks.

Benefits of Active Surveillance

Active Surveillance offers several notable advantages for individuals with low-risk prostate cancer:

1. Avoidance of Treatment Side Effects: One of the primary benefits is the avoidance of potential side effects associated with prostate cancer treatments, such as surgery, radiation therapy, and hormone therapy. These side effects can include urinary incontinence, erectile dysfunction, and bowel issues.

2. Preservation of Quality of Life: Active Surveillance allows individuals to maintain their quality of life without the immediate disruption caused by cancer treatments. This can be particularly important for older individuals or those with significant health concerns.

3. Reduced Overtreatment: Active Surveillance reduces the risk of overtreatment, sparing individuals from unnecessary interventions for a disease that may never progress to a clinically significant stage.

4. Option to Delay or Avoid Treatment: If cancer shows signs of progression during Active Surveillance, individuals can still pursue curative treatments at a later stage. Alternatively, some may opt to continue surveillance if the disease remains indolent.

5. Psychological Well-Being: Active Surveillance can alleviate the psychological burden associated with a cancer diagnosis, as individuals do not face the immediate pressures of treatment decision-making and the associated anxieties.

6. Cost Savings: By avoiding unnecessary treatments and their associated costs, Active Surveillance can lead to substantial healthcare cost savings.

Challenges and Considerations

While Active Surveillance offers significant benefits, it is not without challenges and considerations:

1. Risk of Progression: The primary concern with Active Surveillance is the potential for the cancer to progress to a more aggressive stage over time. Regular monitoring and follow-up are essential to detect any signs of progression promptly.

2. Anxiety and Uncertainty: Living with untreated cancer can be emotionally challenging, and some individuals may experience anxiety or uncertainty about the disease's future course.

3. Compliance and Follow-Up: Active Surveillance requires consistent compliance with monitoring and follow-up appointments, which may be challenging for some individuals.

4. Treatment Decision Timing: Deciding when to transition from Active Surveillance to active treatment can be complex and may vary based on individual factors.

5. Psychological Support: Individuals on Active Surveillance may benefit from psychological support to address the emotional aspects of living with untreated cancer.

6. Limited Data on Long-Term Outcomes: While Active Surveillance has been studied extensively, there is still limited long-term data on its outcomes, especially for younger individuals.

Active Surveillance is a well-established and evidence-based approach to managing low-risk prostate cancer. It offers a prudent alternative to immediate treatment, allowing individuals to avoid treatment-related side effects while monitoring the disease's progression closely. By adhering to regular monitoring and follow-up, individuals on Active Surveillance can make informed decisions about potential treatments if the disease shows signs of progression.

The suitability of Active Surveillance as a management strategy should be determined through shared decision-making between the individual and the healthcare provider. Factors such as age, overall health, cancer characteristics, and individual preferences should guide treatment decisions.

Ultimately, Active Surveillance empowers individuals with low-risk prostate cancer to take a proactive yet cautious approach to their disease, preserving their quality of life while maintaining the option for curative treatment if necessary.

Radiation Therapy in Prostate Cancer

Advances in medical science have led to various treatment options, and radiation therapy stands as a cornerstone in the management of this disease. In this comprehensive guide, we will explore the role of radiation therapy in prostate cancer treatment, examining its principles, techniques, benefits, potential side effects, and the evolving landscape of radiation therapy in prostate cancer management.

Radiation therapy has emerged as a critical treatment modality for prostate cancer, offering curative potential while preserving quality of life. It utilizes high-energy radiation to target and destroy cancer cells within the prostate gland. The selection of radiation therapy as a treatment option depends on several factors, including the cancer's stage, the individual's age and overall health, and the individual's preferences.

Principles of Radiation Therapy

Radiation therapy is based on the principle of selectively damaging cancer cells while minimizing harm to surrounding healthy tissue. The primary goals of radiation therapy in prostate cancer treatment are:

1. Tumor Control: Radiation therapy aims to target and eliminate cancer cells within the prostate gland, preventing further cancer growth and spread.

2. Preservation of Quality of Life: Radiation therapy seeks to minimize treatment-related side effects and preserve the individual's urinary, sexual, and bowel function.

3. Minimization of Harm to Healthy Tissues: Advanced radiation techniques are designed to spare nearby critical structures, such as the bladder and rectum, from radiation exposure as much as possible.

Radiation therapy can be delivered using external beam radiation therapy (EBRT) or brachytherapy, both of which have distinct approaches and considerations.

External Beam Radiation Therapy (EBRT)

EBRT is a commonly used form of radiation therapy for prostate cancer. It involves the delivery of high-energy radiation beams from outside the body to the prostate gland. Key points about EBRT include:

1. Intensity-Modulated Radiation Therapy (IMRT): IMRT is a sophisticated EBRT technique that allows for precise targeting of the tumor while minimizing radiation exposure to healthy tissues. It uses computer-controlled adjustments of radiation intensity.

2. Image-Guided Radiation Therapy (IGRT): IGRT involves real-time imaging during treatment sessions to ensure accurate targeting of the prostate, particularly when daily setup variations can occur.

3. Stereotactic Body Radiation Therapy (SBRT): SBRT delivers a highly focused and potent dose of radiation in a shorter treatment course (usually five sessions or fewer). It is suitable for select low-risk and intermediate-risk cases.

4. Proton Therapy: Proton therapy is a type of EBRT that uses proton particles instead of traditional X-rays to target the tumor. It offers precise targeting and may reduce radiation exposure to surrounding tissues.

Brachytherapy

Brachytherapy, also known as internal radiation therapy, involves the implantation of radioactive sources directly into or near the prostate gland. There are two main types of brachytherapy for prostate cancer:

1. Permanent Seed Implant (LDR Brachytherapy): In LDR brachytherapy, tiny radioactive seeds are permanently implanted into the prostate gland. Over time, the radiation emitted by these seeds treats the cancer cells while minimizing radiation exposure to nearby tissues.

2. High-Dose Rate Brachytherapy (HDR Brachytherapy): HDR brachytherapy involves the temporary placement of a radioactive source within the prostate. The source is typically inserted for a short duration, allowing for precise delivery of a high radiation dose.

Combination Therapies

In some cases, radiation therapy may be used in combination with other treatment modalities to enhance its effectiveness. Common combinations include:

1. Androgen Deprivation Therapy (ADT): ADT, also known as hormone therapy, aims to reduce the levels of male hormones (androgens) that fuel prostate cancer growth. It is often used in conjunction with radiation therapy, especially for intermediate and high-risk cases.

2. External Beam Radiation Therapy (EBRT) with Brachytherapy: This combination, known as dose-escalated radiation therapy, combines the precision of EBRT with the localized treatment of brachytherapy. It is suitable for select intermediate and high-risk cases.

3. Chemotherapy: In advanced or metastatic prostate cancer, chemotherapy may be added to radiation therapy to enhance tumor control.

Benefits of Radiation Therapy in Prostate Cancer

Radiation therapy offers several advantages as a treatment option for prostate cancer:

1. Curative Potential: Radiation therapy has the potential to cure localized prostate cancer, especially in low-risk and some intermediate-risk cases.

2. Preservation of Quality of Life: Radiation therapy aims to minimize treatment-related side effects and preserve urinary and sexual function. Modern radiation techniques, such as IMRT and IGRT, contribute to this goal.

3. Non-Invasive: Radiation therapy is a non-invasive treatment that does not require surgical incisions. This can result in a shorter recovery time and reduced post-treatment pain.

4. Outpatient Treatment: Most radiation therapy sessions are conducted on an outpatient basis, allowing individuals to return home after each session.

5. Shorter Treatment Courses: Advanced radiation techniques like SBRT offer shorter treatment courses, typically completed in one to five sessions, reducing the overall treatment duration.

6. Localized Treatment: Radiation therapy precisely targets the prostate gland, minimizing damage to surrounding healthy tissues.

7. Option for Salvage Therapy: In cases of cancer recurrence after initial treatment (e.g., surgery), radiation therapy may be used as salvage therapy to target residual cancer cells.

Potential Side Effects and Considerations

While radiation therapy offers numerous benefits, it may also be associated with potential side effects and considerations:

1. Urinary Symptoms: Some individuals may experience urinary symptoms during and after radiation therapy, including frequency, urgency, and burning. These symptoms are often temporary but can be managed with medication.

2. Bowel Symptoms: Radiation therapy can lead to bowel symptoms, such as diarrhea or rectal urgency. These symptoms are usually temporary and can be managed with dietary changes and medications.

3. Erectile Dysfunction: Radiation therapy can affect sexual function, leading to erectile dysfunction. The risk varies based on individual factors, and options for managing this side effect include medications, vacuum erection devices, and penile implants.

4. Fatigue: Radiation therapy may cause fatigue, which can vary in intensity. Adequate rest and physical activity can help manage fatigue.

5. Skin Irritation: Some individuals may experience skin irritation or redness in the treatment area, similar to a mild sunburn. Proper skin care can alleviate these symptoms.

6. Long-Term Effects: Radiation therapy may have long-term effects on the bladder and rectum, including an increased risk of radiation-induced cancers in these organs. However, the absolute risk is generally low.

7. Cognitive Impact: Some individuals may experience cognitive changes, often referred to as "brain fog," during radiation therapy. These changes are typically temporary.

Evolving Landscape of Radiation Therapy

The field of radiation therapy for prostate cancer continues to evolve, with ongoing research and technological advancements. Some notable developments include:

1. Advanced Imaging: Improved imaging techniques, such as multiparametric MRI and PSMA-PET, enhance the accuracy of prostate cancer diagnosis and treatment planning.

2. Radiation Dose Escalation: Dose-escalation strategies, including SBRT and high-dose-rate brachytherapy, aim to increase the radiation dose to the tumor while minimizing side effects.

3. Proton Therapy: Proton therapy, which uses proton particles instead of traditional X-rays, is gaining attention for its potential to reduce radiation exposure to nearby organs.

4. Immunotherapy: The combination of radiation therapy with immunotherapy is being explored as a potential way to enhance the body's immune response against cancer cells.

5. Focal Therapy: Emerging approaches like focal therapy target only the areas of the prostate affected by cancer, sparing healthy tissue. These techniques are still under investigation and not widely adopted.

Radiation therapy plays a vital role in the comprehensive management of prostate cancer. It offers curative potential, preserves quality of life, and continues to evolve with technological advancements and research findings. The selection of radiation therapy as a treatment option should be based on a thorough assessment of the individual's cancer characteristics, overall health, and preferences, and it should be made through shared decision-making with the healthcare team.

While radiation therapy may be associated with potential side effects, modern techniques and supportive care measures have significantly reduced their impact. The goal of radiation therapy in prostate cancer treatment is to provide effective cancer control while minimizing treatment-related burdens, allowing individuals to maintain their quality of life throughout their cancer journey.

Hormone Therapy in Prostate Cancer

Prostate cancer management requires a multifaceted approach, and hormone therapy, also known as androgen deprivation therapy (ADT), stands as a pivotal component of treatment. In this comprehensive guide, we will delve into the role of hormone therapy in prostate cancer management, examining its principles, types, mechanisms of action, benefits, potential side effects, and emerging trends in the field.

Hormone therapy, or androgen deprivation therapy (ADT), is a central treatment modality for prostate cancer. It aims to control the disease by reducing the levels of male hormones, specifically androgens, in the body. Androgens, such as testosterone, fuel the growth of prostate cancer cells. By depriving these cells of androgens, hormone therapy effectively inhibits their growth and spread.

Principles of Hormone Therapy

The fundamental principle of hormone therapy in prostate cancer management is to disrupt the androgen signaling pathway, which is crucial for the growth and survival of prostate cancer cells. This is achieved through several mechanisms:

1. Suppression of Testosterone: Hormone therapy reduces the levels of testosterone, the primary androgen, in the body. This is typically accomplished by inhibiting the production of testosterone in the testes.

2. Blocking Androgen Receptors: Some hormone therapies work by preventing androgens from binding to their receptors on prostate cancer cells. This interference disrupts the signals that drive cancer cell growth.

3. Adjuvant Therapy: In certain cases, hormone therapy may be used in combination with other treatments, such as radiation therapy or surgery, to enhance their effectiveness.

Types of Hormone Therapy

Hormone therapy for prostate cancer can take various forms, including:

1. Luteinizing Hormone-Releasing Hormone (LHRH) Agonists: These drugs, such as leuprolide (Lupron) and goserelin (Zoladex), lower testosterone levels by suppressing the production of luteinizing hormone (LH), which, in turn, reduces testosterone production by the testes.

2. Luteinizing Hormone-Releasing Hormone (LHRH) Antagonists: These medications, such as degarelix (Firmagon), directly block the action of LH, leading to a rapid reduction in testosterone levels.

3. Anti-Androgens: Anti-androgens, including bicalutamide (Casodex) and enzalutamide (Xtandi), work by blocking the androgen receptors on prostate cancer cells, preventing them from receiving and responding to androgen signals.

4. Combination Therapy: In some cases, a combination of an LHRH agonist or antagonist and an anti-androgen may be used to maximize androgen suppression.

5. Surgical Castration: Surgical removal of the testicles, known as orchiectomy, is a permanent form of androgen deprivation that reduces testosterone levels.

Benefits of Hormone Therapy in Prostate Cancer

Hormone therapy offers several significant benefits as a treatment option for prostate cancer:

1. Tumor Shrinkage: Hormone therapy can cause a reduction in the size of the prostate tumor, alleviating urinary symptoms and providing symptom relief.

2. Disease Control: For many individuals, hormone therapy effectively controls the progression of prostate cancer, preventing or delaying the spread of the disease to other parts of the body.

3. Palliation of Symptoms: Hormone therapy can provide relief from cancer-related symptoms, such as bone pain, urinary obstruction, and spinal cord compression.

4. Adjunct to Other Treatments: Hormone therapy is often used in combination with other treatments, such as radiation therapy or surgery, to enhance their effectiveness.

5. Downstaging for Surgery: In some cases, hormone therapy may be used to shrink the tumor before surgery, making it more manageable and potentially increasing the likelihood of complete removal.

Potential Side Effects and Considerations

While hormone therapy offers numerous benefits, it is associated with potential side effects and considerations:

1. Hot Flashes: Hot flashes, similar to those experienced by menopausal women, are a common side effect of hormone therapy. They can be managed with lifestyle changes and medications.

2. Sexual Dysfunction: Hormone therapy can lead to sexual side effects, including erectile dysfunction, loss of libido, and shrinkage of the testicles.

3. Osteoporosis: Reduced testosterone levels can increase the risk of osteoporosis, a condition characterized by weakened bones. Bone health should be monitored, and preventive measures may be recommended.

4. Cardiovascular Effects: Hormone therapy may increase the risk of cardiovascular events, such as heart attacks and strokes, especially in individuals with pre-existing cardiovascular risk factors.

5. Metabolic Changes: Hormone therapy can lead to metabolic changes, including weight gain, increased cholesterol levels, and insulin resistance. Monitoring and management of these changes are essential.

6. Emotional and Psychological Impact: Hormone therapy can have emotional and psychological effects, including mood swings, irritability, and depression. Psychosocial support can be beneficial.

7. Long-Term Use: The long-term use of hormone therapy may increase the risk of more severe side effects, such as osteoporosis and cardiovascular events.

Emerging Trends in Hormone Therapy

The field of hormone therapy in prostate cancer continues to evolve, with ongoing research and the development of novel therapies. Some notable emerging trends include:

1. Next-Generation Anti-Androgens: New anti-androgen medications, such as enzalutamide and apalutamide, have shown efficacy in advanced prostate cancer and are being investigated in various clinical settings.

2. Immunotherapy: Immunotherapy approaches, such as immune checkpoint inhibitors, are being explored in combination with hormone therapy to enhance the body's immune response against prostate cancer cells.

3. Biomarker-Driven Therapy: Advancements in molecular and genetic profiling are leading to personalized approaches in hormone therapy, allowing for more targeted and effective treatments.

4. Intermittent Therapy: Some individuals may benefit from intermittent hormone therapy, where treatment is given in cycles, allowing for periods of testosterone recovery. This approach can help manage side effects.

5. Androgen Receptor Targeting: New drugs that target androgen receptors in different ways are being developed and tested, offering potential alternatives for individuals who develop resistance to standard therapies.

Hormone therapy, or androgen deprivation therapy (ADT), is a central pillar in the management of prostate cancer. It plays a crucial role in controlling the disease, providing symptom relief, and improving overall survival. The selection of hormone therapy as a treatment option should be based on a thorough assessment of the individual's cancer characteristics, overall health, and preferences.

While hormone therapy may be associated with potential side effects, including hot flashes, sexual dysfunction, and metabolic changes, modern approaches aim to mitigate these effects and improve the overall quality of life for individuals undergoing treatment. The ongoing research and development of novel therapies and treatment strategies continue to advance the field of hormone therapy, offering hope for improved outcomes and enhanced patient care in the future.

Ultimately, hormone therapy represents a vital tool in the fight against prostate cancer, offering individuals a chance for effective disease control and an improved quality of life.

CHAPTER FIVE

Real-Life Experiences: Overcoming Prostate Cancer Without Surgery

Prostate cancer is a formidable adversary, affecting millions of men worldwide. When faced with a prostate cancer diagnosis, individuals often confront a myriad of treatment options, with surgery being one of them. However, not all prostate cancer journeys necessitate surgery. In this in-depth exploration, we delve into real-life experiences of individuals who have successfully navigated and overcome prostate cancer without resorting to surgery. These stories illuminate the diverse paths and strategies that have enabled them to manage and conquer this formidable disease.

Surgery, in the form of radical prostatectomy, has long been a standard treatment for prostate cancer, particularly in cases where the disease is localized and considered curable. However, surgery is not the only viable option, and in many cases, it may not be the most suitable one. Non-surgical approaches, such as active surveillance, radiation therapy, and various forms of systemic therapies, have gained prominence as effective strategies for managing prostate cancer without the need for surgery.

In this exploration, we will hear from individuals who have chosen non-surgical routes to overcome prostate cancer. Their experiences and journeys shed light on the diverse paths that one can take when faced with this diagnosis.

John's Story: Navigating the Decision for Active Surveillance

John, a 68-year-old retired engineer, received a prostate cancer diagnosis during a routine check-up. His PSA levels were slightly elevated, and a biopsy revealed low-risk prostate cancer with a Gleason score of 6. After discussing treatment options with his healthcare team, John opted for Active Surveillance.

"I was hesitant about surgery because I didn't want to risk the potential side effects," John recalls. "My urologist assured me that Active Surveillance was a reasonable choice given my cancer's characteristics. It felt like a weight off my shoulders to avoid surgery."

John underwent regular check-ups, including PSA tests and digital rectal examinations, to monitor his prostate cancer's progression. Over the years, his PSA remained stable, and repeat biopsies showed no significant changes. John continued with his active lifestyle, enjoying golf outings with friends and spending quality time with his grandchildren.

"Choosing Active Surveillance allowed me to maintain a sense of normalcy in my life," John shares. "I didn't want to disrupt my routine with surgery, and I'm grateful that my cancer has remained stable."

John's experience with Active Surveillance demonstrates that for some individuals with low-risk prostate cancer, close monitoring can be a viable and effective strategy without the need for surgery.

Michael's Journey: Navigating Radiation Therapy

Michael, a 59-year-old school teacher, received a prostate cancer diagnosis after experiencing urinary symptoms and an elevated PSA level. His biopsy results revealed localized prostate cancer with a Gleason score of 7. Michael discussed treatment options with his radiation oncologist and chose external beam radiation therapy (EBRT).

"I was concerned about the potential side effects of surgery, especially given my profession as a teacher," Michael explains. "I didn't want to risk urinary incontinence or prolonged recovery time."

Michael underwent a course of EBRT, which involved daily sessions for several weeks. During treatment, he continued to work and maintained an active lifestyle. Although he experienced some fatigue and mild urinary symptoms during treatment, these side effects gradually improved after radiation therapy was completed.

"After completing radiation therapy, I felt relieved that I didn't have to go through surgery," Michael reflects. "I'm back to my regular activities, and my follow-up PSA tests have shown a decline."

Michael's experience illustrates how radiation therapy can be a viable and effective alternative to surgery, allowing individuals to maintain their daily routines and minimize treatment-related disruptions.

David's Battle: Navigating Systemic Therapies

David, a 63-year-old business executive, faced a challenging journey with prostate cancer. His initial treatment with radiation therapy did not completely eradicate the cancer, and his PSA levels continued to rise. Further imaging tests revealed the presence of cancerous lesions in his bones, indicating advanced disease.

"I was devastated by the news of my cancer's progression," David shares. "I knew surgery wasn't an option at this point, and I needed a different approach."

David's oncologist recommended hormone therapy, also known as androgen deprivation therapy (ADT), to target the androgens fueling his cancer's growth. Hormone therapy aimed to suppress testosterone levels, which are known to drive prostate cancer.

"While hormone therapy isn't a cure, it's been effective in slowing down the cancer's progression," David explains. "I've also explored new treatments, such as immunotherapy, as part of clinical trials. These therapies give me hope."

David's journey highlights the importance of systemic therapies in managing advanced prostate cancer when surgery is no longer a viable option. While it may not provide a cure, systemic therapy can offer valuable time and opportunities for individuals to explore emerging treatments and clinical trials.

Robert's Holistic Approach: Integrative Prostate Cancer Management

Robert, a 70-year-old retiree, adopted a holistic approach to managing his prostate cancer. After receiving a low-risk prostate cancer diagnosis, he chose Active Surveillance as his primary strategy. Simultaneously, he incorporated lifestyle changes into his daily routine.

"I felt that I had an active role to play in managing my health," Robert explains. "I started by revamping my diet, focusing on whole foods, and reducing processed sugars."

Robert also embraced regular exercise, incorporating walking and yoga into his lifestyle. He attended mindfulness and meditation classes to reduce stress and anxiety associated with the cancer diagnosis.

"I believe that the mind and body are interconnected," Robert says. "Mindfulness helped me cope with the emotional aspects of cancer, and yoga improved my flexibility and overall well-being."

Robert's integrative approach to prostate cancer management illustrates the importance of addressing both physical and emotional aspects of the disease. Integrative strategies can complement conventional treatments and enhance an individual's overall quality of life.

Prostate cancer is a complex and multifaceted disease that presents individuals with a range of treatment options. While surgery has been a traditional approach, it is not the only path to overcoming prostate cancer. Through the real-life experiences of individuals who have successfully navigated prostate cancer without surgery, we have explored the diversity of strategies available.

Active Surveillance, radiation therapy, systemic therapies, and integrative approaches all have their place in the spectrum of prostate cancer management. Each individual's journey is unique, shaped by factors such as cancer characteristics, personal preferences, and overall health.

The experiences shared here remind us that there is no one-size-fits-all solution to prostate cancer. The decision-making process should involve open communication with healthcare providers, a comprehensive understanding of treatment options, and careful consideration of individual circumstances. Prostate cancer can be managed successfully without surgery, allowing individuals to pursue the path that aligns best with their values, goals, and quality of life.

Collaborating with Your Healthcare Team in Prostate Cancer

In this comprehensive guide, we will explore the critical importance of collaborating with your healthcare team in prostate cancer management. We'll discuss the roles of various healthcare professionals, the process of shared decision-making, the significance of clear communication, and how teamwork can lead to more informed and personalized treatment choices.

Collaboration with your healthcare team involves actively engaging with a group of healthcare professionals who work together to provide comprehensive care, tailored to your unique needs and preferences. These professionals may include urologists, radiation oncologists, medical oncologists, nurses, radiologists, pathologists, and more. Their collective expertise and teamwork play a pivotal role in guiding you through the diagnosis, treatment, and survivorship phases of prostate cancer.

Building Your Healthcare Team

Your journey in managing prostate cancer begins with assembling a knowledgeable and supportive healthcare team. Each member of this team contributes a specific set of skills and expertise to ensure the best possible care. Here are some key players you may encounter:

1. Urologist: Often the first point of contact, urologists specialize in diseases of the urinary tract and male reproductive system. They can diagnose prostate cancer, discuss treatment options, and perform surgeries if necessary.

2. Radiation Oncologist: Radiation oncologists specialize in radiation therapy, a crucial treatment option for prostate cancer. They work to develop and implement radiation treatment plans tailored to your specific case.

3. Medical Oncologist: Medical oncologists specialize in cancer treatment using medications, such as chemotherapy, hormone therapy, and targeted therapies. They manage systemic treatments and address advanced cases.

4. Nurse Navigator: Nurse navigators are experienced nurses who guide you through the healthcare system, providing information, support, and assistance with coordinating appointments and care.

5. Pathologist: Pathologists analyze biopsy samples to determine the type, grade, and stage of prostate cancer. Their findings help guide treatment decisions.

6. Radiologist: Radiologists interpret imaging tests, such as MRI and CT scans, to assess the extent and location of prostate cancer. Their reports aid in treatment planning.

7. Dietitian: Dietitians provide guidance on nutrition and diet during and after treatment. They help manage side effects and promote overall well-being.

8. Psychologist or Social Worker: Psychologists and social workers offer emotional support, counseling, and resources to help you cope with the psychological and social aspects of prostate cancer.

The Importance of Shared Decision-Making

Shared decision-making is a cornerstone of patient-centered care. It involves a collaborative process in which you, as the patient, work closely with your healthcare team to make informed treatment decisions. The goal is to tailor treatment plans to your preferences, values, and unique circumstances. Shared decision-making typically involves the following steps:

1. Understanding Your Diagnosis: Your healthcare team should explain your prostate cancer diagnosis in clear, understandable terms. This includes details such as cancer stage, grade, and risk factors.

2. Exploring Treatment Options: Your team should present all available treatment options, including surgery, radiation therapy, hormone therapy, and active surveillance. They should discuss the potential benefits, risks, and side effects of each option.

3. Evaluating Personal Preferences: You and your healthcare team should discuss your personal preferences, priorities, and quality-of-life considerations. These factors can greatly influence treatment decisions.

4. Setting Realistic Expectations: Your team should help you understand what to expect during treatment, including potential side effects and recovery times. Realistic expectations are crucial for informed decision-making.

5. Making a Decision: Once you've gathered all the necessary information and had thorough discussions with your healthcare team, you can make an informed treatment decision. It's essential that you feel comfortable with the choice you make.

6. Follow-Up and Reevaluation: As your treatment progresses, your healthcare team should continually assess your response and adjust the treatment plan as needed. Regular follow-up visits are crucial for monitoring your progress.

Effective Communication with Your Healthcare Team

Clear and effective communication is vital in ensuring that you receive the best possible care for prostate cancer. Open dialogue with your healthcare team fosters trust, facilitates shared decision-making, and helps address concerns as they arise. Here are some communication strategies to consider:

1. Prepare Questions: Before appointments, write down any questions or concerns you have about your diagnosis, treatment options, or side effects. This will help ensure that you cover all relevant topics during your visit.

2. Actively Listen: Pay close attention to what your healthcare team is saying. If something is unclear or you need further clarification, don't hesitate to ask for more information.

3. Speak Up: Be proactive in sharing your thoughts, preferences, and feelings with your healthcare team. Your input is invaluable in tailoring your care plan.

4. Keep a Record: Maintain a record of your medical history, including test results, treatment dates, and medications. This can help you and your healthcare team track your progress.

5. Engage Family Members: If you wish, involve a family member or close friend in your healthcare discussions. They can provide support and help ensure that nothing is overlooked during appointments.

6. Seek Second Opinions: It's entirely appropriate to seek a second opinion from another healthcare provider, especially when facing significant treatment decisions. A fresh perspective can offer valuable insights.

7. Utilize Online Resources: Reliable online resources, such as reputable cancer organizations and medical journals, can provide additional information and support for your journey.

Multidisciplinary Tumor Boards

Multidisciplinary tumor boards are meetings where healthcare professionals from various specialties come together to review and discuss complex cancer cases. These boards ensure that you receive the benefit of multiple expert opinions when making treatment decisions.

Tumor boards are particularly valuable in cases of advanced or complex prostate cancer. They provide a forum for urologists, radiation oncologists, medical oncologists, radiologists, pathologists, and other specialists to collectively evaluate your case and develop a comprehensive care plan.

Survivorship and Follow-Up Care

Survivorship care is an essential component of prostate cancer management. After completing treatment, regular follow-up visits with your healthcare team are crucial to monitor your progress, manage side effects, and address any potential recurrence or complications.

Survivorship care may also include addressing quality-of-life concerns, such as sexual function, urinary continence, and emotional well-being. Rehabilitation and support services can help individuals regain their full range of physical and emotional health.

Collaborating with your healthcare team is fundamental in prostate cancer management. By building a strong healthcare team, engaging in shared decision-making, fostering effective communication, and utilizing multidisciplinary tumor boards, you can navigate the complex landscape of prostate cancer with confidence.

Remember that you are not alone on this journey. Your healthcare team, along with the support of loved ones, can provide the guidance and expertise you need to make informed decisions and achieve the best possible outcome in your battle against prostate cancer.

Future Trends and Emerging Treatments in Prostate Cancer

While current treatment options have advanced over the years, researchers and healthcare professionals continue to explore innovative strategies to improve outcomes and enhance the quality of life for individuals with prostate cancer. In this exploration, we will delve into the future trends and emerging treatments in prostate cancer, offering insights into promising areas of research and potential game-changers in the field.

The management of prostate cancer has evolved significantly, with a range of treatment options available, including surgery, radiation therapy, hormone therapy, and chemotherapy. However, the complexity of the disease and its varied clinical behaviors necessitate ongoing research and innovation to optimize treatment outcomes and reduce side effects.

Future trends and emerging treatments in prostate cancer encompass a broad spectrum of approaches, from precision medicine and immunotherapy to novel imaging techniques and targeted therapies. These advancements aim to address the diverse needs of individuals with prostate cancer and offer hope for improved survival and quality of life.

1. Precision Medicine and Genomic Profiling

Precision medicine, also known as personalized medicine, is a rapidly advancing field that tailors treatment to an individual's genetic makeup and the specific characteristics of their cancer. In prostate cancer, genomic profiling is playing a pivotal role in guiding treatment decisions.

Genomic profiling involves analyzing the genetic mutations and alterations present in a patient's cancer cells. This information helps identify potential therapeutic targets and predicts how a patient may respond to specific treatments. Genomic profiling has the potential to:

- Identify Targeted Therapies: By pinpointing genetic alterations, such as mutations in the BRCA genes, precision medicine can guide the use of targeted therapies that specifically attack cancer cells while sparing healthy tissue.

- Personalize Hormone Therapy: Genetic profiling can inform the selection of hormone therapy options, ensuring that individuals receive the most effective treatment based on their unique genomic profile.

- Predict Treatment Response: Genomic profiling can help predict how a patient's cancer will respond to certain treatments, allowing for more informed treatment decisions and potentially avoiding ineffective therapies.

- Identify Clinical Trials: Patients with specific genetic mutations may be eligible for clinical trials testing novel therapies that target those mutations.

2. Immunotherapy

Immunotherapy is a groundbreaking approach that harnesses the body's immune system to recognize and attack cancer cells. While immunotherapy has shown remarkable success in various cancers, its application in prostate cancer is an emerging area of interest.

One promising avenue in prostate cancer immunotherapy is the use of immune checkpoint inhibitors. These drugs, such as pembrolizumab (Keytruda) and nivolumab (Opdivo), block specific proteins that cancer cells use to evade the immune system. Early clinical trials have demonstrated encouraging results, particularly in individuals with advanced prostate cancer who have limited treatment options.

Another exciting development is personalized cancer vaccines. These vaccines are designed to stimulate the immune system to recognize and target the unique antigens present on cancer cells. While still in the experimental stages, personalized cancer vaccines hold promise for prostate cancer treatment.

3. Radiopharmaceuticals and Targeted Alpha Particle Therapy

Radiopharmaceuticals are radioactive substances that can be combined with specific molecules to target and deliver radiation directly to cancer cells. In prostate cancer, radiopharmaceuticals are increasingly being used for both diagnostic and therapeutic purposes.

One notable radiopharmaceutical is ^{177}Lu-PSMA-617, which targets prostate-specific membrane antigen (PSMA), a protein highly expressed on prostate cancer cells. This radiopharmaceutical is used in a form of targeted alpha particle therapy known as radioligand therapy. It has shown promise in clinical trials for individuals with metastatic castration-resistant prostate cancer (mCRPC), offering a new treatment option when other therapies have failed.

Radiopharmaceuticals not only provide a targeted approach to treatment but also offer a non-invasive way to assess disease progression through molecular imaging techniques like PSMA-PET scans. This enables more accurate staging and monitoring of prostate cancer.

4. Focal Therapy and Ablative Techniques

Focal therapy is an emerging approach that targets only the specific areas of the prostate affected by cancer, sparing healthy tissue. This technique is particularly relevant for individuals with localized prostate cancer who wish to minimize treatment-related side effects.

Focal therapy methods include high-intensity focused ultrasound (HIFU), cryotherapy, and laser ablation. These techniques precisely deliver energy to destroy cancer cells while leaving the surrounding tissue unharmed. Focal therapy is still undergoing research and development, and its long-term effectiveness is being studied. It offers the potential for curative treatment with reduced risk of urinary incontinence and erectile dysfunction compared to traditional radical treatments.

5. Advanced Imaging and Early Detection

Improvements in imaging technologies are transforming the early detection and monitoring of prostate cancer. Multiparametric magnetic resonance imaging (mpMRI) and PSMA-PET scans are enhancing the accuracy of prostate cancer diagnosis and staging.

MpMRI combines multiple imaging techniques to provide detailed images of the prostate gland, helping identify suspicious areas for targeted biopsies. PSMA-PET scans, which use a radioactive tracer that binds to PSMA on cancer cells, offer a more sensitive and specific method for detecting and locating prostate cancer, especially in cases of recurrent or metastatic disease.

These advanced imaging techniques aid in better characterizing the extent and aggressiveness of prostate cancer, facilitating more precise treatment planning and monitoring.

6. Combination Therapies

The future of prostate cancer treatment may lie in combination therapies that utilize multiple approaches simultaneously or sequentially. For example:

- Combining radiation therapy with immunotherapy is being explored as a way to enhance the immune response against prostate cancer cells.

- Combining targeted therapies with chemotherapy or hormone therapy may improve treatment outcomes, particularly in advanced or treatment-resistant cases.

- Sequential therapies, where different treatments are administered in a specific order, are being investigated to maximize treatment effectiveness while minimizing side effects.

Combination therapies aim to exploit the synergistic effects of various treatments to achieve better disease control and patient outcomes.

7. Lifestyle Interventions and Supportive Care

While medical treatments continue to advance, lifestyle interventions and supportive care remain essential components of prostate cancer management. Diet and nutrition, exercise, stress management, and psychological support play crucial roles in improving the overall well-being and quality of life for individuals with prostate cancer.

- Diet and Nutrition: A balanced diet rich in fruits, vegetables, and whole grains can support overall health and may help mitigate treatment-related side effects.

- Exercise and Physical Activity: Regular exercise can improve physical fitness, reduce fatigue, and enhance emotional well-being during and after treatment.

- Stress Management: Techniques such as mindfulness, meditation, and counseling can help individuals cope with the emotional challenges of a prostate cancer diagnosis.

- Supportive Care: Support groups, patient advocacy organizations, and counseling services provide invaluable support and resources for individuals and their families.